TANGLES

AND

PLAQUES

A MOTHER AND DAUGHTER
FACE ALZHEIMER'S

SUSAN CUSHMAN

eLectio Publishing

Little Elm, TX

www.eLectioPublishing.com

Tangles and Plaques: A Mother and Daughter Face Alzheimer's
By Susan Cushman

ISBN-13: 978-1-63213-340-3
Published by eLectio Publishing, LLC
Little Elm, Texas
http://www.eLectioPublishing.com

Printed in the United States of America

5 4 3 2 1 eLP 21 20 19 18 17

The eLectio Publishing creative team is comprised of: Kaitlyn Campbell, Emily Certain, Lori Draft, Court Dudek, Jim Eccles, Sheldon James, and Christine LePorte.

Publisher's Note
The publisher does not have any control over and does not assume any responsibility for author or third-party websites or their content.

Dedicated to the memory of
Effie Watkins Johnson
(1928-2016)

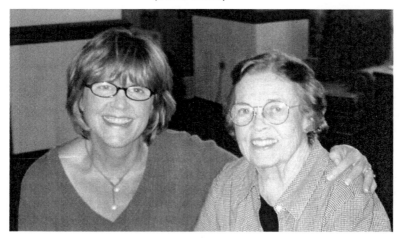

**(Photo taken on Mother's Day 2007,
the year I wrote my first blog post about our relationship)**

More praise for *Tangles and Plaques*

"Susan Cushman writes with clarity and grace about the gnarled pathways between her and her mother, and about the terrible disease that holds a surprising grace within its irrevocable sadness. *Tangles and Plaques* has the courage to see it all. This is a memoir about caretaking and taking care. It's a book that will touch your heart."

—Lee Martin, author of
From Our House and *Such a Life*

"An honest, open account of the personal challenges, wrenching heart aches, spiritual questions, and practical concerns one faces in caring at a distance for a loved one with Alzheimer's. Cushman provides intimate, detailed descriptions of her constant doubts, emotional upheavals, hard decisions, and frustrating encounters with professional caregivers during the decade of the unrelenting progression of her mother's mental and physical deterioration."

— Sally Palmer Thomason, author of
The Living Spirit of the Crone: Turning Aging Inside Out,
The Topaz Brooch, and
Delta Rainbow-the Irrepressible Betty Bobo Pearson.

"Susan Cushman writes a profoundly personal and honest portrait of her eight-year journey with her mother suffering from Alzheimer's. She brings her talent for story, scene, and character to bear in the unfolding of real-time moments that show disease progression and the ensuing softening in a challenged relationship. Cushman sees and feels things deeply and finds in each encounter a nugget of wisdom that fortifies her with focus, peace, and faith. Her stories give inspiration and insight to others who face this journey."

— Kathy Rhodes, author of
Remember the Dragonflies: A Memoir of Grief and Healing

"*Tangles and Plaques* is a beautiful and moving memoir and one that chronicles the journey of Alzheimer's. Through the tangles and plaques associated with the disease, however, Cushman finds a way to heal and set her sight on the good. Readers, too, get a lesson in how to live better."

—Niles Reddick, Vice Provost,
The University of Memphis-Lambuth,
and author of *Drifting Too Far from the Shore.*

You say "Thank you" when something scary has happened in your beloved and screwed-up family and you all came through (or most of you did), and you have found love in the intergenerational ruins (maybe a lot of love or maybe just enough).

—Anne Lamott,
Help, Thanks, Wow: The Three Essential Prayers

The upside of Alzheimer's: new mother.

—Susan Cushman,
Smith's Six-Word Memoirs

CONTENTS

The New Epistolary

In the seventeenth and eighteenth centuries, epistolary novels—based on letters or journal entries by one or more characters—were all the rage. In today's social media culture, blog posts have upstaged journal entries and letters. A collection of those posts could be called the new epistolary.

On November 24, 2007, I wrote my first blog post about my mother, Effie Johnson, and her journey with Alzheimer's. Over the next eight and a half years, I published a total of sixty posts about Mom. With very little editing, those posts now appear as essays in this collection. I chose to treat these posts like letters of the past; each one becomes a spot in time in the ever changing landscape in the life and relationship of an individual woman, my mother, and her daughter.

Why "Tangles and Plaques"?

The title comes from my blog post of August 13, 2012. Here's an excerpt:

The brain has 100 billion nerve cells (neurons) that operate like tiny factories. Alzheimer's disease prevents parts of a cell's factory from running well. As the disease spreads, cells lose their ability to do their jobs and eventually die, causing irreversible changes in the brain.

With this loss of brain cells comes the loss of memory—the stories that make up the fabric of a person's life—as well as the inability to perform everyday life chores.

Tangles and plaques tend to spread through the temporal lobe cortex and hippocampus as Alzheimer's progresses.

Neurofibrillary tangles are twisted fibers of another protein called tau, which build up inside the cells.

Argyrophilic plaques are deposits of a protein fragment called beta-amyloid, which build up in the spaces between nerve cells.

Shortly after this book was accepted for publication, Mom passed away. I'm so glad that she is done with the tangles and plaques, and has joined my father—her spouse of 49 years—on the other side, because the quality of her life after eight years in a nursing home—being fed through a PEG tube to her stomach since January of 2013—was certainly not what I desired for her.

My close friends and relatives know that loving Mom and caring for her has been complicated by her emotional and verbal abuse of me (and my brother) for most of my life. Those issues are addressed in several of the blog posts comprising this book. The silver lining in Mom's disease is that the same tangles and plaques that stole most of her memory also erased the dysfunctional part: she forgot how to criticize and abuse. In her altered state, she was much easier to love. To forgive.

I live in Memphis and Mom was 200 miles away in Jackson, Mississippi. During these years as I blogged about my long-distance caregiving, I have received many positive comments from readers, some of whom are also in the position of caring for a parent with Alzheimer's. It was an easy decision to gather these stories into a book so that I could share them with more readers. Not wanting to lose the immediacy and voice, each original blog post was written within a day or two after my visit with my mother.

I have tried to blend humor ("The Glasses," "I Can't Find My Panties") with pathos ("Disappearing Stories," "End of Life Issues")—hope with despair—in these essays. Alzheimer's is a universal issue, especially for those of us in the generation tagged the "Baby Boomers."

According to the Alzheimer's Association, the disease is "the only cause of death among the top ten in America that cannot be prevented, cured, or slowed." It is the sixth leading cause of death in the United States. One in three seniors dies with Alzheimer's or another form of dementia, and more than fifteen million people provide care to people with dementia.

Mom is second generation Alzheimer's. Her mother died with the disease at age 86—in the same nursing home where my mother lived. Of course I watched my mother's decline with fear and trembling. I often saw myself in her place, and all I can do is pray for God's mercy, and for a breakthrough in the research being done to try to stop this modern-day plague. It is my hope that my mother's journey—and mine—will resonate with readers who share these struggles. I think you will find that the tangles and plaques aren't only in our brains, but often in our relationships.

Piece of Mind
Saturday, November 24, 2007

My mother's name is Effie Johnson. She has Alzheimer's. At age 79 she's been on meds for over five years and has been a resident at an assisted living home in Jackson, Mississippi, for almost two years. Ridgeland Pointe specializes in memory loss. After a few weeks in her new home her mind seems better, possibly because her meds are managed by the nurses, and she is taking them regularly for the first time. And because her world has become smaller. More manageable. The people at Ridgeland Pointe seem to really care about her. Which gives me much peace of mind.

I visit Mom about once a month (I live 200 miles away in Memphis) and of course I can see the gradual decline. My husband went with me to see her on Thanksgiving Day. It was the first time he'd seen her since my brother's funeral back on February 1. So the change was much more noticeable to him. It's not just her memory that's being destroyed by this awful disease; it's how she functions in the present, as well. Even when we're having a good time, like during our visit to a coffee shop on Thanksgiving afternoon, there seems to be a fog moving in, covering her mind, making it hard for her to see out and for us to see in. I had to cut through that fog to explain what the pastries were in the bakery counter at the coffee shop—muffins and scones and cookies and cakes. She stood there for a long while just pointing at everything in the case and saying, "How pretty!" She couldn't grasp the idea that these were edible items and she needed to choose something, so I ended up ordering for her.

So, yesterday when I met up with some friends at the Brooks Museum of Art (back in Memphis) for the Pissarro show, I was really more anxious to see the exhibit of artwork done by some of the participants at the Alzheimer's Day Services of Memphis. The exhibit was called "Piece of Mind." Karen Peacock, an art therapist, helped the participants with their work. My friend Julie Stanek

5

was with me Friday. She teaches art at Rossville School and is working on her Master's at Memphis College of Art. In fact, she's working on a project dealing with art therapy right now.

Of course it made me wish my mother could participate in an activity like this. She has lots of talent, but hasn't painted since her college days, where she minored in art. I've always admired her artsy handwriting and decorative touches on gifts. One Christmas back in the '60s my father and brother and I gave her a set of oil paints as a gift, hoping she would start painting again. But she always thought she was too busy for what might have seemed like a leisurely pursuit. Instead she busied herself with substitute teaching, garden club, bridge club, luncheon club—all more acceptable activities for a Southern woman in the 1950s. I'm going to send information about the program to her assisted living facility director in hopes that they can find an art therapist to work with the residents, to help them get in touch with parts of themselves that are slipping away. To give them an outlet for their creativity.

It's not that I don't have peace of mind about Mom's care where she is. It's a wonderful place. It's just that this exhibit made me want more for her. All the years she was too busy being a school teacher—and then a full-time mom and substitute teacher, and later a small business owner with my dad—she set aside her own creative impulses to take care of her children and later to support my dad in his dream of running an athletic retail business and organizing community running events. They owned Bill Johnson's Phidippides Sports in Jackson, Mississippi, from 1982-1997. Dad also ran many marathons, including Boston and New York quite a few times, while he was in his 60s. Mom was always in his shadow, a loyal supporter.

So now I'm thinking maybe it's Mom's turn. I hope she'll have a chance to paint.

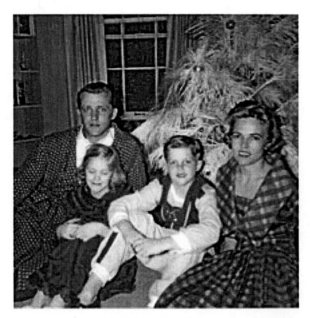

Christmas Eve 1959
Dad, me, Mike and Mom

She Can't Possibly Be Eighty, Because...
Friday, February 22, 2008

Mother can't be eighty, because that would mean that I'll be fifty-seven in a few weeks. But what's all this ado about age, anyway? This is really about mothers. And daughters. And birthdays.

I went to Jackson yesterday to celebrate my mom's 80th birthday. I was going to give her a party, but she asked me not to. And when I got to her assisted living home early Wednesday afternoon, the staff had just celebrated her birthday at lunch with cake and balloons and everything. But she didn't remember. Alzheimer's is like that, even in the early stages.

But she was happy to see me. And she loved the blouses and slippers I took her. She has become more focused on colors and textures lately. She also enjoyed the chocolates that my friend Sue gave her. Sue drove me down so I could keep my foot propped up in the backseat since it still tends to swell when it's not elevated. (I'm recovering from surgery on my left foot.) We took Mom for an outing.

First we drove around our old neighborhood so I could show Sue and Mom the house we built when I was seven. I think Mom recognized it. And the school I went to from second through sixth grades, which is about four houses down from our house. We drove up and down the streets of our old neighborhood. I pointed out the houses where our best friends lived. The McCreights. The Sumralls. The Coxes. Mom seemed to remember their names, but she's getting to the point where she will try to cover for her memory loss. I think she's embarrassed.

Then we took her to Starbucks for lattes. Later we picked up some wine and shared a toast with her at her apartment and said goodbye. Looking in from the outside, she might seem like a fully functioning person. But I could see the storm clouds gathering.

On our drive back to Memphis, Sue asked me about my childhood, and we talked about mothers and daughters. Recently a friend told me that she was really close to her grandparents because her parents were too much into their own drama to pay attention to her. This is kind of like what Kim Sunee says in her book, *Trail of Crumbs*, about her adoptive mother, who was too self-absorbed to care about her. Kim, too, was drawn to her grandparents, who seemed to want to spend time with her. My kids could probably say the same about me. God forgive me.

Maybe it's just the nature of the generations. While mothers are too busy trying to find themselves, grandmothers bond with their children. I don't remember my mother being self-absorbed, but she was verbally abusive to me for many years. She was obsessed with my weight and the way I dressed and wore my hair. Always criticizing me. But I was really close to her mother, "Mamaw." When I got home today I got out some photo albums and looked at pictures from my childhood, looking for clues.

I found this one, taken on Christmas Eve 1959. God, my mother was beautiful. She was 31. I've got on my new red silk nightgown and robe. My brother, Mike, and my dad have on their jammies. And then there's Mom, dressed to the nines and looking like a movie star. I think we had just come home from church and she hadn't changed clothes yet.

She's still beautiful. And now she takes me around her assisted living home and introduces me to everyone as her "little girl." And she smiles her movie star smile. She doesn't criticize me as much as she used to. I'm hoping those tendencies are getting lost in the fog.

I just kiss her and tell her I love her. Happy birthday, Mom.

The Glasses
(previously published in
Southern Women's Review, January 2010)
Thursday, April 17, 2008

"I just can't get my glasses clean." Mom was riding with me to do some shopping when she pulled her glasses off and held them up to the windshield for a better view of the smudges.

"Here, I've got a special cloth for cleaning lenses," I offered.

She fumbled with the cloth for a few minutes. At a stoplight, I took the glasses and tried to clean them for her.

"Mom, these are all scratched up... in fact, these are your old glasses. Where are the new ones we got you?"

"Oh, I think they fell under my bed."

"Well, when we get back to your apartment, I'll look for them."

"Oh, no. You couldn't possibly fit under the bed. There's only a tiny, tiny space there."

"But I could at least see if they're there, and maybe fish them out with a yardstick or something."

"No, there just isn't room under that bed, I promise you."

"Well, I'll still look for them when we get back."

After shopping we went to lunch. Trying to read the menu, Mom took her glasses off and said, "These glasses are so dirty, I can't see a thing through them."

"That's because they're scratched, Mom, remember? I'm going to look for your new glasses when we get back to your apartment."

"Oh, don't worry about it. I'm sure they'll turn up some time."

After lunch, I took her to get a manicure and pedicure. Sitting across from her and reading fashion magazines while a cute guy did her nails, I realized we'd been together for three hours, and I hadn't asked her any of the questions I'd been thinking about from my childhood. They'd have to wait 'til we got back to her place now. Or I could just listen as she entertained the employees and other customers at the nail place.

"This is my little girl." She pointed to me. "She lives in Memphis. She took my car away and sold my house. But she comes to visit me about once a year."

I smile at the young women in the chairs next to her, fighting back the urge to defend myself. One of them gives me a knowing wink, which helps. And then the young man doing Mom's nails says, "Now, Mrs. Johnson, your daughter brought you in here just a month ago to get your nails done, didn't she?"

"Oh, I don't know. She lives in Memphis. *Ouch!*"

"Sorry, I didn't realize your toe was tender."

"Well, it is. Something's wrong with it. I've been meaning to get someone to look at it."

The nail on the big toe of her right foot was thick and green with fungus.

"Mom, I took you to the doctor last month and she told us what to do about it. Remember? I got you some Vicks VapoRub to put on it twice a day. I wrote you a note and taped it to the Vicks bottle by your bed. Have you been putting it on your toe?"

The giggles the other customers had been trying to stifle just couldn't be held in any longer at this. So I said to the room, "I know it sounds ridiculous, but Mom's internist told us that more than one of her patients has had success with this."

A few minutes later, as we're leaving the nail place, with Mom wearing a pair of free, disposable flip-flops, she looks at her feet and says, "What's wrong with the nail on that big toe?"

"You've got a fungus, Mom."

"Oh. Is there anything we can do about it?"

"We can try putting Vicks VapoRub on it. I've got some for you back at your apartment."

"Vicks? Really? Well, I'll try anything once!"

Back in the car, we're driving through a neighborhood that had been hit by tornadoes a couple of weeks ago. Mom says, "I think I saw this on the news, but I didn't realize how bad it was."

"Me, either. Wow—look at that huge tree completely uprooted over there. And all those houses with blue tarps on the roofs where trees fell on them. My goodness."

At this Mother took off her glasses and held them up to the window. "I can't really see them well. My glasses are so dirty. Do you have something I can clean them with?"

"We already cleaned them, Mom. They're scratched. Those are your old glasses. We need to find your new ones when we get back to your apartment."

"What new ones?"

"The ones you think might have fallen under your bed."

"Oh, don't worry about it, these are fine."

Back at Ridgeland Pointe, Mom's assisted living facility, we make our way through the lobby, where she "introduces" me to all her friends. Again. Finally we're back in her apartment and I'm on my hands and knees looking under her bed for the glasses.

"You can't see anything under there, Susan. The space is just too small."

"I can see fine, Mom, but there's nothing under here."

Up off my knees, I begin to search her bedside table, and finally the bookcase headboard behind her pillow.

"Here they are, Mom!"

I hand her the glasses, and she looks at them, then at me, and says, "Oh. I like my old ones better. But thanks, anyway."

The Good Daughter
Thursday, June 12, 2008

"Mrs. Cushman? Is this Effie Johnson's daughter?" The weekend nurse was calling me on my cell phone from my mother's assisted living home in Jackson, just as Katherine and Daphne and I were enjoying our last hour together in the car on the drive home from the Yoknapatawpha Writers Workshop in Oxford.

"Yes, this is Susan Cushman. Is something wrong?"

"Yes, ma'am. Your mother is real upset with me and I don't know what to do."

"Just a minute, please." I turned to Daphne and Katherine, who were continuing to break down all the juicy details of the weekend, and said, "Please wait 'til this phone call is over. I really don't want to miss a word!"

Silence fell over the car and I continued to talk with the nurse.

"Her eyes are red and itching something awful, and even her cheeks are red and patchy and irritated. One of the other residents tried to give Miss Effie some of her prescription eye drops and I told her, 'No, ma'am, those are yours and could hurt Miss Effie's eyes and I could lose my license!'"

"Is Bobbye there?" I've become friends with the regular nurse, but I didn't recognize this voice.

"No, ma'am, just me."

"And what's your name?"

"I'm Mary."

"Okay, well hi, Mary. I think you're doing everything you can. Do you think I should call Mother's doctor this afternoon and get her to call in some drops, or do you think she'll be okay if we wait until tomorrow, since today's Sunday and it's already 5 p.m.?"

"Oh, I think she'll be fine until tomorrow. I'll leave a note for Bobbye to call you in the morning."

"Thanks, Mary. Oh, and you can tell Mother that you talked to her daughter and we're going to get her some drops."

"Yes ma'am. She and the other lady are really mad at me."

"Well, the good news is that she won't remember that she's mad at you tomorrow, or even later today. She might not even remember who you are since she has dementia."

In the two years Mom has been in assisted living, I've rarely received phone calls from a nurse, so I was afraid it was a real emergency. Once I realized that nothing needed to be done until tomorrow, I joined back into the conversation with my friends.

We had only about an hour left to decompress a three-day workshop! Funny how "real life" seems to intrude on our creative efforts.

Three days later I drove back down to Jackson to see Mom, after talking with the nurse on Monday and learning that she got the drops from Mom's doctor and was already administering them, along with a special cream for her face. Mom's friends are always glad to see me when I walk in the door, though. I'm greeted with, "Oh, Susan, I'm so glad you're here. Your mother won't quit rubbing her eyes and her face is all broken out and her eyes are itching and burning and…."

Like I can control Mother's behavior. Over the next five or six hours, as we visited in her apartment, at Starbucks, and eventually at Le Nails, I probably reminded her fifty times to quit licking her fingers and rubbing her eyes and her cheeks with her spit. Bless her heart, they are bright red and burning.

"Ooooooooh," she whined like a child, "please don't fuss at me. They itch."

"I know they itch, Mother, but you are making them worse licking your fingers and rubbing off the medicine from your cheeks with your spit and then rubbing it into your eyes."

"I am *not* doing that."

Times fifty.

So I got a plan: I'd take her to get a manicure, so her fingers would be "busy" for at least a half hour or so. Once we got to Le Nails, I decided to let her get a pedicure as well, while I got my nails done at another chair.

Mom climbed up onto the oversized recliner and put her feet into the hot, bubbly water. Like a queen on her throne, she had a view of everyone in the room:

Three women and one man were working on four to six clients, with two more waiting.

Mom surveyed the room, looked at me, then swept the room with a loud voice as she said, "This is my little girl. She lives in Memphis."

One or two people glanced in my direction and I smiled, subtly.

"She doesn't come to see me very often," was Mother's next proclamation.

With that, I received several sympathetic looks, especially from the nail techs, who knew us from previous (and frequent) visits. But one woman who missed the nod to me following the first comment looked at my mother and said, "Oh, how often does she come and visit you?"

Mother hesitated, a confused, glazed look covered her face, and before she could speak, I raised my hand from across the room to get the woman's attention.

"Uhm, that would be me—I'm the daughter," I said, meekly, and then added, "I visit about once a month."

I spared the woman the back story—how I also do all of Mom's finances, file her income taxes, buy all her clothes and personal items for her, and send her handwritten cards, letters and photos between my monthly visits. I am a good daughter. So, why do I feel guilty, no matter how much I "do" for Mother? Before I could finish that thought, Mom started back up again.

"Yes, she's my little girl. But she ate too much, and now she's my BIG girl."

I felt a dozen eyes on my hips and thighs at that moment, and I thought about explaining that I had foot surgery in January and haven't been able to exercise and I've gained some weight but I plan to get back to exercising soon and hope to lose the weight because, well, because I'm a good daughter.

Earlier that day we had been in line at Starbucks behind a rather large black woman when Mother pointed to the woman's butt, puffed her cheeks up with air and raised her eyebrows. I put my finger to my lips to shush her and prayed that she wouldn't say anything aloud.

I repeated the prayer later at Le Nails when a chubby young teenage girl walked in with her dad. They arrived in time to hear the comment about my eating too much and getting big. I hope no one ever tells that little girl that she is fat. She knows, and she'll deal with it how and when and if she wants to or is able to at some point. I just hope someone loves her unconditionally. It looks like she's got a sweet daddy, who brought her in for a manicure and pedicure. And got one himself—yes, he was a manly man, too.

As Mother and I prepared to leave Le Nails, I hurried to pay for our manicures and pedicures, hoping to escape more embarrassing comments from Mom. The nail tech who took my money smiled at both of us and said to me, "Thank you for coming and bringing your mother in today."

Before I could reply, Mother smiled back at him and said—loudly enough for everyone in the salon to hear—"She's a good daughter."

I picked up my receipt and as I looked down to put it in my purse, tears dropped onto the paper, smearing the ink, blotting out the bad memories, at least for a moment.

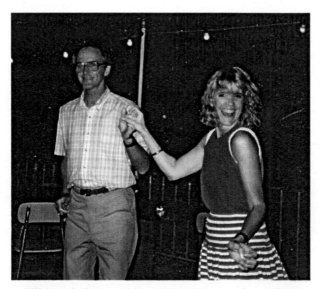

**Bill (my father) and Susan dancing on a houseboat
on the Ross Barnett Reservoir, Jackson, Mississippi, 1988**

The Good Daughter, Part II
Saturday, July 12, 2008

It's been an emotional week. July 9 was the ten-year anniversary of my father's death, and July 11 was the ten-year anniversary of his burial. He was only 68, a strong, healthy marathon runner whose life was cut short by cancer. The photo on the previous page is me and Dad in the late '80s, probably just a year or so before we moved to Memphis, dancing on a houseboat on the Ross Barnett Reservoir at a party for employees at the business he and my mother owned for fourteen years, Bill Johnson's Phidippides Sports.

Today was my monthly visit with my mother at the assisted living facility. It's hard to decide, when caring for someone with progressive dementia/Alzheimer's, how much to try to micro-manage the domestic and personal care issues they can no longer carry out. I'm really trying to let her live in peace, without spending every minute of our visits together picking up the pieces of her life that she continues to drop. For example, for several months now I've been ignoring the growing pile of clothing that now covers half her bed. She continues to pull clothes out of drawers and off hangers in her closet, trying to decide what to wear, what things need cleaning, what she doesn't want anymore, etc. I've offered to help with the process several times, but she's always declined the offer in the past, choosing instead to go out on excursions in the car, like shopping and lunch. But today she was tired and wanted to stay in, so I started in on the pile of clothes.

"Those clothes aren't dirty."

"Mom, they even smell bad."

"I can't smell anything."

"Look at the food stains."

"Oh—those won't come out. They wouldn't come out the last time I washed them."

But I persisted and eventually she just sat on the half of the bed not covered with clothes and watched as I sorted things into piles to be washed or given away.

The laundry room is just down the hall, so I loaded up three machines with her clothes and then went to work on the stacks of newspapers and trash in the sitting area of her apartment. She allowed me to carry these out to the trash without argument, which cleared a spot where I could sit with her and watch the birds on her birdfeeder outside her window.

"Look! There's my redbird! I just love to watch the birds."

"Did Ken [the maintenance man] help you put up the new column of food?"

"Yes, just the other day. I could sit here for hours—the view is so pretty. Look at the clouds." Mom has always been into clouds. I think her inner artist sees more than meets the eye.

I try to stay in the moment, but I can't help noticing that her hair hasn't been washed in a while and her fingernails are chipped and ragged.

"Did you get your hair done this week?"

"No. I just didn't feel like it." The beauty parlor is in the building. But it's not open on Saturdays.

"Would you like me to take you to someone out in town and get a perm today?"

"No, I'll get them to do it here one day soon. It's really not bothering me. Look! The cardinal just came back!"

Okay, this is good. She's letting go of menial concerns and enjoying the important things. I could learn something here. So I try to relax and just visit while making runs back and forth to the laundry room to hang up blouses and slacks and fold undershirts. Suddenly it's noon and I ask if she'd like to go out for lunch.

"No. Let's just eat here today. It's too hot to go out in the car." It was really steamy, so I agreed.

The dining room has tables for four, and Mom has three regular tablemates, so we pull up a fifth chair for me at her table. Her best friend, Elizabeth, has been such a good companion for Mom since she moved in two and a half years ago. Although she has physical problems and needs a walker to get around, Elizabeth has always struck me as having a sharp mind, so she and Mom kind of balance each other out. Until today.

While we were waiting for Jamie, a regular at the table who is younger and very clear-thinking, Elizabeth starts giving me *her* take on Jamie:

"The woman who sits next to me has Alzheimer's, but she doesn't know it. We never know what she's talking about. She just goes on and on about things, and she doesn't know she has Alzheimer's."

"Jamie?" I'm astounded. I glance at Mom for a response, but she's looking off somewhere else in the dining room and not paying attention to Elizabeth's words.

"Yes," Elizabeth insists. "They brought her here and asked me to watch after her, but I told them I'm not equipped to do that, that she's too far gone. And besides, I'm already responsible for the cats."

How could I have been so wrong about Elizabeth's state of mind? Elizabeth has two cats in her tiny apartment, and she feeds the feral cats who live behind the building. She's had open heart surgery and both her legs swell, which is why she uses a walker. And of course, she's not responsible for Jamie, or anyone else.

Jamie joins us and I find myself paying more attention to her, being sure I wasn't wrong that she's the one who's still in her right mind. First she wheels another resident to her table (in a wheelchair) and tells her she'll be back after lunch to help her. Then she greets me by name and asks about my family, clear as a bell. She proceeds to tell me what's wrong with her eyes and how difficult it's been to have to give up driving. Her two sons live in town, which is a big help. Very clear words. Another resident stops

23

by our table and reminds Jamie of their date to play Scrabble at two o'clock. Jamie is definitely alert.

Next Elizabeth begins to point at another woman who is pushed into the room in a wheelchair a few tables away.

"Look, she's back. Poor thing. She was born without any legs and you would think the doctors could find some appliance that would help her, but she's just been to a convention where they display all the latest things and they didn't have anything that would work for her."

I look over at the woman and I'm speechless. It's Bernice, the mother of a close friend of mine from high school. She had a stroke just over a year ago and moved into Ridgeland Pointe. I've been visiting with Bernice each month when I go to see Mom, but I noticed she wasn't there last month.

Did I mention she has both legs?

She was in the hospital for six weeks—another stroke. She has an aide helping her eat, as she's lost more control of her arms than before. But she's in good spirits. We have a nice chat and then I return to my mother's table.

Mother and Elizabeth are finishing their desserts and Elizabeth is filling several containers with leftover cornbread, rice and lima beans for the cats. I guess they're vegetarians, but I don't ask. I've already heard more than I can process from Elizabeth today, so we say goodbye for a while and head back towards Mom's apartment. But first we stop off at the laundry room to get her clean clothes.

As I'm folding the last of the clothes, Mom begins stroking her clean blouses and *talking to them*, saying, "Oh, I'm so sorry she put you in those machines and got you all wet. You were just fine the way you were. I tried to tell her so."

"Mom, can't you just say 'thank you for washing my clothes' and be happy that they're so fresh and clean now?"

"They weren't dirty."

"Well, they're clean now."

24

"But they weren't dirty."

Sigh. We took them to her apartment, hung up the blouses and slacks and put the other items into the drawers by her bed. It occurred to me that she might have a hard time finding them, since she's been used to them being on the bed, so I labeled the drawers with sticky notes and carefully showed her where the blouses and slacks were, after moving the winter clothes to the far end of the closet. It all looked so fresh and neat and made *me* feel so good.

"It looks strange in here," was all she could say.

We visited in the sitting area for a while again, and finally I said, "Would you like to go somewhere?"

"Like where?"

"We could go to Starbucks... and maybe to Le Nails for a manicure and pedicure?"

"Okay."

That was easy. We got our drinks at Starbucks, then drove to the nail salon and walked in to find there would be a thirty-minute wait, so we sat in the waiting area, looking at magazines and picking out nail colors. Having a nice outing, or so I thought.

But as the minutes ticked by, Mom became agitated.

"It's hot in here."

The air conditioning seemed fine to me.

"Do I really have to do this?"

"Why wouldn't you want to, Mom? It's been a month since you had your nails done, and you used to do this every week, remember?"

"Did I? Was it always so hot?" Now she's pulling her shirt off her shoulders and fanning herself with a magazine. Then she begins whining: "Please, I don't want to. Can't you just take me home? *Please!*"

"Okay, sure." I let the technicians know we'll come back another day and I help Mom to the car. It's ninety-something degrees, of course, but compared to the air-conditioned nail salon, Mom seems to like it.

"I just didn't feel like doing that today."

"That's fine, Mom. I just thought it would make you feel better to have your nails done. But we'll do it next time," and then I add, *"if you want to."*

She perks up during the drive back to her apartment, and again I point out familiar landmarks from the sixty years she's lived in Jackson. As we pass a small red building I ask her, "Do you remember what that building is, Mom?"

"No."

"It's your dentist's office. I haven't taken you there in over a year, because you said you didn't want to go anymore. You had some crowns done that will hopefully help you keep your own teeth so you won't have to get dentures. But I could take you to have your teeth cleaned some time if you'd like me to."

She opens her mouth in a Garfield smile to expose her top and bottom teeth and says, "Look, my teeth aren't dirty."

"Like your clothes aren't dirty?" I ask.

She just nods and smiles.

I'm learning.

Once we're inside the lobby of her assisted living facility and she sees some of the other residents, she's happy again.

So it's come to this. Her world is getting smaller and her concern for things like hair and teeth and fingernails and clothing is dwindling. But her interest in birds and clouds and trees is growing. Yes, the disease of Alzheimer's is eating away at her mind. But she's still a person, created in the image of God. As I finish these reflections tonight, I remember the words of Jesus, "Whoever does not receive the kingdom of God as a little child will by no means enter it."

Maybe she's closer to the Kingdom than I am. And not just because she's eighty.

The Good Granddaughter
Monday, August 4, 2008

My daughter Beth and I drove down to Jackson to visit my mom this weekend. Beth hadn't seen her in a while 'cause she's been busy with grad school (architecture at UT Knoxville) so I tried to prepare her for the decline in my mother's mental condition. Her memory loss seems to be hastening a good bit in the past few months, but thankfully her temperament has improved. Most of the time she's pretty happy, and she tells me over and over how much she likes her assisted living home now. She's been there two and a half years. I think it took her about a year and a half to really make the shift from grieving the loss of her house and independence to contentment in her new situation. Which is pretty admirable, actually.

Anyway, the last time I was there I noticed that all the photographs I send her were beginning to pile up around her apartment, covering the window ledges and other areas that needed to be dusted but couldn't be seen. So I bought her a bulletin board and packed it, and a few tools, for our trip down. We picked up some salads from the Beagle Bagel and took them to Mom's apartment just before lunch so we could eat with her while we worked on the bulletin board, instead of eating in the dining room like I did last time.

While we're eating lunch, Mom asks Beth, "What are you doing these days, Beth?"

"I'm in graduate school, studying architecture. And working."

"Oh, that's exciting. I guess that keeps you busy."

"Yes ma'am."

And then she asks me about the boys and I tell her that Jon is home from Iraq safely and then I remind her that Jason got married in May and show her the picture of him and his wife again and she says they're a cute couple and then she asks Beth, "So what have you been doing this summer?"

"I'm in school and working."

"In school? What are you studying?"

"Architecture."

"Oh, that sounds exciting."

After four or five more rounds of this conversation, we are finished with lunch and start working on the bulletin board.

Granny Effie watches while Beth reads the instructions and then attaches the hangers to the back of the bulletin board. "What are you doing?"

"She's fixing your bulletin board so we can hang it on the wall," I answer, leaving Beth free to keep working.

"What for?"

"So we can put all your pictures up there so your window seat and end table won't be so messy."

"They don't bother me."

"I know, Mom, but you'll enjoy them more this way, and when I send you more pictures you'll have room for them."

"My bird feeder is empty."

"Yeah, I forgot to bring more bird food this trip."

"I love to sit here and look out this window. It's so pretty. But the bird feeder is empty."

"We'll get some more soon, Mom. Would you like to go out with me and Beth and get some today, when we're finished with the bulletin board?"

"What are you going to do with the bulletin board?"

"We're going to arrange your pictures on it, like this—"

"Oh, that's nice. But I really need a manicure."

"Yeah, I'm sure you do. A few weeks ago when I took you to the nail place you changed your mind and asked me to bring you home, so you didn't get one that day."

"Can you do my nails for me?"

"No, I don't have all the right stuff, Mom, but they can do your nails in the beauty parlor upstairs here. Do you want me to make you an appointment?"

"No, I'm not in the mood."

Beth has finished with the hardware and is ready to arrange the pictures, so I gather up the stacks and start selecting a few for her to group together.

"Here—put some captions with each group to remind Mom who folks are and what was going on in each picture."

Granny Effie gets up to watch Beth arranging the pictures and looks out the window, where a big yellow machine is parked next to the building, with a crane reaching up to the roof.

"They're working on our building," she says.

I look and see roofing materials.

"Oh, that must be roof repairs from the tornadoes that came through here a couple of months ago. I'm glad they're fixing the roof. Although I feel sorry for the men working on the roof today—it's over 100 degrees!"

About then Beth has finished arranging the photographs and we hang the bulletin board on the wall.

Mom beams. "Oh, I love it. Can I go see if Elizabeth wants to come see it?"

"Sure, Mom."

Elizabeth comes over and loves the bulletin board. Then she sits down to visit with us, and begins telling us about her cats.

"My big tom cat is named Rosey. I named him after Roosevelt Grier, the football player, because he's huge."

"That name sounds familiar." I look at Beth, who always knows sports trivia. "Who did he play for?"

"Some team in California," Elizabeth begins. "He was the only good one in the whole bunch of them. And he was huge."

Beth gets out her new phone and Googles Roosevelt Grier and sure enough he played for the Los Angeles Rams in 1972 and his nickname was "Rosey."

"Yes, he was a good man. He quit playing football and became a preacher."

Beth verified this info from her phone and added, "And he did needlepoint and he knitted."

About then one of the aides came in the door looking for Elizabeth. "Mrs. McKay, I've got your antibiotic. I thought you'd be over here with Miss Effie when I couldn't find you in your room."

"Oh, where is it?"

The aide hands the pill and a cup of water to Elizabeth, who takes the pill and then looks out the window and says, "There's that big girl who works here, Emily? Just sitting out on the patio. What's she doing out there? She's so big and she's just sitting out there."

I look out the window. "That's one of the construction workers taking a break from working up on the roof, Elizabeth."

"No, that's that fat girl that works here. She is so big."

About then the aide giving Elizabeth her pill says, "Now, I bet you talk about me like that when I'm not here." This aide has lots of braids, dyed red, and pulled up on top of her head so that they stick out in all directions. "I'll bet you say, 'There goes that big girl whose hair looks like it's on fire' or something like that." And the aide starts laughing. Mom and Beth and I are cracking up by now.

Elizabeth says, "I'm sure that's that big girl out there on the patio."

I look again. "That's a Hispanic *man* sitting there, Elizabeth."

"Well, I can't see very good anymore."

We won't have time to take Mom out to buy birdseed unless we leave soon, and just as I'm about to suggest we leave, Elizabeth starts back up.

"I've got a friend who is Chinese. Her parents are pure Chinese. They came from China. But they know a lot about adoption."

I'm guessing this conversation is sparked by Beth's presence, but I'm not sure, and Elizabeth never addresses Beth directly about being Asian or adopted. She just keeps talking.

"Anyway, I went to a funeral for a family member of hers and it was a genuine Chinese funeral. At the end, they threw a funeral wreath up on the roof of the house. It was all completely Chinese."

"That's an interesting custom, Elizabeth." I try to join the thread. "Are they Buddhist?"

"No, they're Chinese. They're from China."

Mom seems to want to join the conversation but it's hard to find a place to jump in so she says, "I can't tell the difference if someone is from China or Japan. They look the same to me."

Beth and I share understanding looks throughout the visit, and I'm so thankful she's there. She's patient and sweet with Granny Effie and somehow it just helps me for her to be part of the circle.

About then I say it's time for us to be on the road and so Mom and Elizabeth start walking with me and Beth out of Mom's apartment and towards the front of the building. On the way we see one of Mom's dining room tablemates, Jamie, playing Scrabble with another resident. Jamie hugs me and I introduce her to Beth and she hugs Beth and tells her, "We're taking good care of your grandmother." Later I remind Beth that Jamie is the one that Elizabeth thinks has Alzheimer's, but Jamie is the one who plays Scrabble.

On the drive back to Memphis, I tell Beth I'm so glad she came, and thank her for helping me with the bulletin board. Well, actually, she did most of it herself and I just watched. She certainly made my trip to Jackson so much lighter this month. She's a Good Granddaughter.

Unhappy Chairs
Thursday, September 11, 2008

"Mrs. Cushman? This is Kelly. I'm the nurse administrator at your mom's assisted living home. No emergency—but please call me when you can."

The last time I got one of these calls I was driving home from a workshop in Oxford, and the weekend nurse was frantic about Mom's eyes—she had an infection and wouldn't quit rubbing them and her cheeks were inflamed from Mom's continual licking of her fingers and then rubbing them on her cheeks to soothe them. Thankfully, that got taken care of. So when I got the message this time, I assumed it was another urgent, but not serious, health issue. Wrong.

"We've noticed that your mom is slipping in several areas and would like for you to consider moving her to our Alzheimer's unit upstairs where we can take better care of her."

My heart sank. I knew this day was coming, of course. I knew it when I moved Mom into the facility in February of 2006. But she's so happy in her current situation, where she is free to roam about the facility at will—the light, cheerful lobby areas, the front patio with rocking chairs, the back courtyard area where her birdfeeder is, the large atrium dining room, and four wings of apartments. Moving "upstairs" would mean that she would be "locked in" to her wing, with only a screened-in porch at the end for exposure to the outdoors. But it would also mean she would get more help in the areas that she's beginning to need it.

So I made an appointment and drove down to meet with the nurse and marketing director on Tuesday. Well, by the time I got there, things had changed a bit. The nurse and I had agreed over the phone that Mom would do better if she moved about the same time as her best friend, Elizabeth, who really needs to move soon. But Elizabeth was protesting and her family was also a bit resistant, so they're letting her stay downstairs for a while. Probably a few more months. This gave me time to adjust to the idea myself, and to hear about the benefits Mom would receive upstairs, which could really be good for her at this stage of Alzheimer's.

When I finished meeting with the nurse, I went down to Mom's apartment for a visit. When I asked how she's doing she said her back had been hurting. Really her hip, where she's had bursitis for a long time.

"Let's stop by the physical therapy room after lunch and see if they can do something to help you," I suggested.

"Oh, it's not that bad. I don't want to."

As we sat in her living room area, looking out at the courtyard and her bird feeder, I noticed a bunch of chairs huddled together on the back patio.

"What are those chairs doing out there, Mom?"

"Oh, I am so upset. Those are our dining room chairs and they are getting rid of them. I loved those chairs. They are so pretty and comfortable and happy."

"Well, I'm sure the new ones must be nicer or they wouldn't be replacing them."

"Oh, no. They are ugly ugly ugly. They are uncomfortable and unhappy."

"Mom, chairs aren't happy or unhappy. They're just chairs. People can choose to be happy or unhappy, and you can choose to be happy about the new chairs."

"No, it's the chairs that are unhappy. Just wait 'til you see them at lunch."

So, I went to lunch with Mom and as we entered the dining room area I was surprised by how pretty the new chairs were.

"Mom, these are really pretty!"

About then Elizabeth greeted us, and Jamie, another tablemate.

As soon as I sat down Mom said, "Aren't these chairs uncomfortable?"

Jamie said, "I think they're elegant."

"You would," Elizabeth chimed in.

Jamie winked at me. She's the one with the most brain cells still working.

"Mom, chairs aren't people—they don't have feelings. And you can choose how to feel about these chairs, which are lovely."

Our food came, tasty pork tenderloin, turnip greens, rice and gravy, cornbread, fruit and cake. Mom picked at her food as she always does, but eventually ate about a fourth of it. She only weighs about 125 pounds. But she's always loved turnip greens.

"Mom, you're not eating your turnip greens. You used to eat a whole bowl of them with a piece of cornbread for your meal. Don't you like them anymore?"

"I've never really liked turnip greens."

"Sure you did. Remember when you would buy bagfuls of them and wash them in the sink and pick the leaves off the stems and cook them down with fatback for us? They were delicious, especially when you made a skillet of cornbread to go with them."

"No, I don't remember ever liking them. And these chairs are really ugly."

Trying to distract her from the chair issue, I offered to get us some coffee.

"They've moved the coffee stand to way over there at the end of the dining room," Mom started back in. "It used to be right there," she pointed, "close to our table."

"It's only a few feet further away now." It was Jamie, the voice of reason, again. "And besides, we need the exercise." Another wink.

I got our coffee and we finished our cake and finally it was time to say goodbye to the dining room and the unhappy chairs.

On the way back to Mom's apartment, Mom complained about her back hurting again, so we stopped by the physical therapy room so I could meet the new full-time therapist and encourage him to work with Mom. Her lower back and hip were really hurting. Nothing new—her bursitis just kicks up from time to time.

"Oh, I don't want to go in there—they'll hurt me!"

"No they won't, Mom, they'll do some things to help your back pain."

We met the new staff, including Grant, a handsome thirty-something guy with an old-fashioned movie-star quality to fit his name.

"He's cute!" Mom noticed immediately.

"Yes—wouldn't you like to have him help you with your back pain?"

"Will it hurt?"

Grant smiled and offered his hand in introduction. "We won't hurt you, Miss Effie. But we can show you some exercises that will make you feel better."

We looked around the room at some of the other residents they were working with. No one was screaming in pain. Some were even smiling, so I hope Mom will cooperate with them when I'm gone.

Back in the hall near Mom's apartment, we found her friend Elizabeth, sitting on a bench, distraught.

"What's wrong?" I asked as we approached.

"That woman with the ponytail has been telling everyone that I'm moving upstairs to the Alzheimer's unit. Can you imagine that? As though I have Alzheimer's? Dr. Fulcher's nurse just evaluated me last week and couldn't find anything wrong with my brain. They're just spreading rumors."

"We won't let them take you," Mom said, sitting down beside Elizabeth on the bench and putting her arm around her.

I looked for an opportunity to plant some positive seeds.

"The apartments upstairs are just like the ones you have now. And some day, when you both need a little more assistance with things, wouldn't it be nice to move upstairs together?"

Mom actually nodded and seemed to accept the idea. I hope Elizabeth will warm up to it in coming months. They will both get a higher level of personal care up there.

I only hope they have happy chairs.

Oh, and by the away, while looking for pictures of "unhappy" chairs on the Internet, I found a book called *50 Sad Chairs*. Maybe eventually I'll learn not to argue with my mother.

My Mother's Keeper
Thursday, October 23, 2008

After a cruel childhood, one must reinvent oneself. Then reimagine the world.

—Mary Oliver

I've been reading these words, penned by the Pulitzer Prize–winning poet Mary Oliver, over and over lately. Not only because of the things that are stirring in my soul and memory as I continue work on my memoir, but possibly even more so because of the increasing time I am spending with my mother in her physical and mental decline. The words are powerful to me because I believe that my mother might have endured a cruel childhood at the hands of her father, my grandfather. And that same cruelty was perpetrated on me in my early years, also by her father.

Mary Oliver experienced this suffering, and she writes about it in her book, *Blue Pastures*:

> *Adults can change their circumstances; children cannot. Children are powerless, and in difficult situations they are the victims of every sorrow and mischance and rage around them, for children feel all of these things but without any of the ability that adults have to change them.*

What struck me about these words as I read them again this morning is that my mother has become a child again, a victim of Alzheimer's and a broken hip. Helpless as a child in her current circumstances, completely dependent upon the kindness of strangers, family and friends. As her only living child, I am her connection to those sources of kindnesses. *I am my mother's keeper.*

Thankfully, I have help. Comfort Keepers have been providing sitters around the clock for Mom since the day she entered Baptist Hospital, October 8. They have continued to provide help during the weeks Mom has to stay in the rehab section of Manhattan Nursing Home. I've had the joy of getting to know one of those

39

sitters in particular, Sondra, a delightful woman from South Africa. She's been Mom's day sitter for the past couple of weeks, and now Mom thinks she's a friend who also lives in the nursing home with her. Every morning Sondra brings Mom a thermos of fresh coffee from her home, with just the right amount of sugar in it. During the afternoons, while Mom is in physical therapy, Sondra takes the thermos to the dining room at the nursing home and refills it for Mom's afternoon coffee when she returns to her room. She calls me on her cell phone every day and keeps me informed of Mom's progress, and also of her concerns, so that I can address them with the proper people there—sometimes a social worker, sometimes a physical therapist, sometimes a nurse.

Yesterday Sondra said she had a question for me. "Is that large, colorful picture of a parrot on the wall on the other side of her room hers? It's hanging by her roommate's dresser, but your mother is saying it's hers and she's telling me to take it down and bring it to her side of the room."

It's actually a huge jigsaw puzzle of a parrot, surrounded by tropical plants, which has been glued together and hung on the wall. It's the only thing of any color on the other side of the room, where Priscilla lives. Priscilla is older than Mom, and diabetic. I caused a huge stir last weekend when I offered her one of Mom's chocolate candies. The nurses came flying into the room, wrestled them from her as she was screaming, and then scowled at me for giving her the candy. What was I thinking? Of course I had no idea she was diabetic, but now I understand that you never offer food or drink to anyone in a nursing home (or hospital, for that matter) without asking a nurse.

Nor do you help an old lady in a wheelchair onto the elevator. Mom's room is on the second floor, and as I was leaving the building one day last week, a woman was struggling to get herself onto the elevator to go downstairs.

"Can you help me, please?" Her hands were gnarled and curled onto the arms of the wheelchair. Her feet touched the floor, propelling her along the hallway.

"Of course." I smiled cheerfully and held the elevator door open for her. She still couldn't get the chair over the threshold, and just as I began to help her, a nurse came running around the corner. The lady's "alarm" had triggered the nurse. She isn't allowed off the floor. If she had made it downstairs and out the front door, no telling what might have happened.

Again, I listened humbly to the nurse's explanation and apologized. I have so much to learn as we enter this next stage of Mother's life. As humiliating as they were, both experiences gave me confidence in the nursing home's care for its residents, keeping them safe from sugar and strangers. Since Mother can't remember where she is or why she is there most of the time, I'm encouraged by the security in place in the home.

Even when I fought against it at first. When I found they had put Mom in a diaper, I was as upset as Mom was. What an affront to her dignity! She begged me to get her panties for her and to get her out of the diaper.

I charged down to the nurses' station and asked why my mother was in a diaper, when she's perfectly capable of using a toilet.

"Her orders say that she can't put any weight on her legs at all yet. Only a physical therapist can get her in and out of the bed."

"But we have sitters with her 24/7. Why can't they help her?"

"Because they aren't trained to move her in just the right way. Even the nurses aren't allowed to do that yet. If she puts weight on her leg in the wrong way, or falls, she could break her hip again. Once she's done a few days of physical therapy, we'll probably get orders that she can use the bathroom with help."

I tried to explain this to Mother. And sweet Sondra patted her hand and told her she'd leave the room when Mom needs to "go" and then she'll quickly change and clean her. She's allowed to do that since Mom has the strength to hold onto the bed rail and pull herself onto her side. The sitter isn't allowed to turn Mom herself.

A week later Mom is making progress with the therapy and I'm told that she'll be allowed to use the toilet, with the sitter's help, in a day or two. She seems to find this comforting, and asks for something to write down the date so she will know when she can use the toilet. Mom has survived the past five years or so with increasing dementia mainly by writing things down. Come to think of it, that's pretty much how I make it through my day, too.

That and cable TV. I took Mom's small TV from the bedroom of her assisted living apartment to the nursing home last week, and the Comcast cable guy came out on Friday to hook it up. His name was Mike, same as my brother, who died in January of 2007. But Mom didn't seem to associate him with Mike. Instead, she just enjoyed his presence immensely.

"Have we met before?" she asked him.

"Yes. In Paris, back in 1948, I think it was." He didn't miss a beat with his delightful answer.

"Paris?" Mom looked at me. "Have I ever been to Paris?"

"Don't you remember our weekend together?" Mike had her full attention now.

By this time the sitter and I were laughing and Mom started laughing, too, and soon Mike had her cable set up and began asking her what kind of TV shows she liked to watch.

Of course Mom didn't remember, so I helped out, mentioning Atlanta Braves baseball, any football games that involved Peyton or Eli Manning, and old movies. Before we knew it, Mike had programmed several stations that would play these things so that all she had to do was push the "FAV" (favorites) button and it would scroll through those channels. He even included a music channel that played '40s swing music. He clicked it on just in time for an old Benny Goodman number, and he and I started dancing and Mom started swinging her arms in the bed and smiling to the beat of the band.

Yeah, Mike the cable guy is a keeper.

Yesterday the head nurse and marketing director from her assisted living home visited Mom at the nursing home. They were checking on her progress, assessing whether or not she will be able to live in the downstairs/assisted part of Ridgeland Pointe in a few weeks, or whether she'll have to move to the upstairs/Alzheimer's wing. I toured the Alzheimer's wing last week, and I really hope Mom can stay downstairs, where she has the run of the building, with its cathedral ceiling dining room, airy and sunny lobby, and front porch. Evidently Mom has become everyone's sunshine at Ridgeland Pointe, and they all miss her and want her back.

So, Mom was in the living room at the nursing home when Kelly and Erin came to visit. Sondra had taken her down in her wheelchair to hear someone sing, which Mom loves. When Kelly and Erin approached her, she lit up, smiled, and greeted them cheerfully, but soon it became obvious that she had no idea who they were. She sees them every day at Ridgeland Pointe, but she's been away for two weeks. *Sigh.* I hope her lack of memory of them won't be a mark against her. They'll assess her again next week.

Much more to say here, but I'm off to my Memphis Writers' Group's monthly meeting, then driving down to Jackson for a few days. So, this is to be continued. Oh, and my Oxford Writing Group meets Saturday, so I'll spend the day there on my way back to Memphis on Saturday. Framing my days with Mother between these two escapes into the world of creative writing and literature. That's what Mary Oliver did:

> *Whatever can take a child beyond such circumstances, therefore, is an alleviation and a blessing. I quickly found myself two such blessings—the natural world, and the world of writing: literature. These were the gates through which I vanished from a difficult place.*

Oh, I think I hear the siren call of poetry and prose coming from my writing group buddies at Starbucks, and the more distant sound of novels-in-progress wafting up from the Yoknapatawpha Writing Group in Oxford.

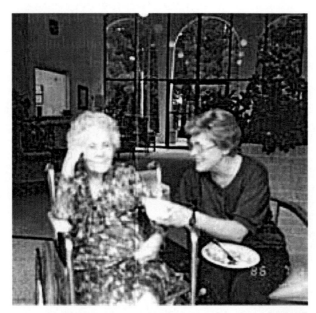

Emma Sue Watkins with her daughter Effie Watkins Johnson
in the lobby at Lakeland Nursing Home,
July 16, 1986, Jackson, Mississippi

Her Mother's Keeper
Sunday, October 26, 2008

When she was my age, my mother was taking care of *her* mother, "Mamaw," at Lakeland Nursing Home in Jackson, Mississippi. The picture on the previous page was taken on Mamaw's 87th birthday, July 16, 1986. Mom was 58, just a year older than I am now. Mamaw died a couple of months later. I'm not sure how many years she was in a nursing home. There weren't special facilities for people with Alzheimer's then, or at least not in Jackson. She never fell and broke her hip like Mom did. The Alzheimer's just gradually shut down her bodily functions.

In 1986 Mom was just recovering from treatments for cancer. That's a wig she's wearing. We've really shared (and survived) a lot of common life experiences.

I remember being angry with her when she first put Mamaw in a nursing home, in the early 1980s. I wanted her to let Mamaw live with her and Dad, not in an institution. How could she do that to her mother?

Those thoughts still haunt me today, as I consider my own mother's future. When I moved her out of her own house and took away her car two and a half years ago, I offered for her to live with us in Memphis. We even bought a house with a downstairs guest suite just for her. But she refused, and begged me to let her stay in Jackson, where she had lived for almost sixty years. That's when I found Ridgeland Pointe Assisting Living. It's a great apartment, and I hope she'll be able to live there again.

When she was ready to leave the hospital after surgery for her broken hip a couple of weeks ago, I was asked which nursing/rehab facility I wanted her taken to. Lakeland (where Mamaw had lived) was my first choice, but there were no female Medicare beds available at the time, so she ended up at Manhattan, which seemed to be an adequate facility. But it's not home. And every time I'm there trying to help Mom deal with her confusion and pain, I look at the faces of so many elderly people in the halls in their wheelchairs and I feel pangs of guilt all over again. Couldn't I take care of her at home, with help from sitters? Isn't that the right thing to do?

But it only takes a few hours with her to remind me of my inadequacies. I'm just not able to endure her pain, emotionally, on an ongoing basis. Or my own pain as her presence reminds me of years of verbal abuse. The sitters have emotional distance, and a great sense of humor, which enables them to possibly be kinder and more helpful. I'm also not capable of the level of physical care she needs now.

Friday afternoon I went upstairs to visit with Mom. A huge banner had been hung on the wall that said *Get Well Soon!! We Miss You!* It was signed by dozens of her friends and staff members at Ridgeland Pointe. The director of nursing and the marketing director from Ridgeland Pointe had come to see Mom the day before and brought the banner to her. The sitter had told me that Mom had no idea who they were when she saw them. And these were two people she saw almost every day for the past two and a half years.

"Oh, Mom! Look at that wonderful banner from your friends at Ridgeland Pointe!"

"What's Ridgeland Pointe?"

"It's the assisted living home, where your apartment is... where you've been living for the past couple of years."

No lights go on. Her expression remains blank, so I continue.

"Remember your best friend, Elizabeth, lives there? That's her, with you in that picture." I point to the picture of the two of them, which I brought from her apartment last week. She and Elizabeth have been inseparable for the past year or two.

"What's her name?"

"Elizabeth."

"Is she still living?"

"Yes, Mom. She lives right across the hall from you at Ridgeland Pointe. She has cats, remember? And you eat at the same table in the dining room three times a day."

Mom points at the door of her nursing home room and says, "Across the hall, here?"

"No, Mom, at Ridgeland Pointe, where you live."

"I don't live here?"

"No, this is just a rehab center where you're doing physical therapy to get your hip well so you can go back home to Ridgeland Pointe."

"What's wrong with my hip?"

This conversation, like many others, was repeated several times during the afternoon. When my patience began to wear thin, and Mom's irritability level rose, I distracted her by asking if she'd like a glass of wine. That seemed to erase the afternoon's arguments, and I unzipped her suitcase in the corner of the room and pulled out one of the small, screw-top bottles of Chardonnay I had stashed there. I poured it over ice (that's how she likes it, unless it's really cold already) and handed it to her and sat down beside her. As she sipped, she noticed again the "things" on her roommate's bureau, which she thinks belong to her.

"Those are my things over there. She stole them from me."

"No, Mom, those are Priscilla's things. You have your own ice pitcher and flowers and stuff—just look at all these things you have!"

I poured a small cup of wine for myself and tried to draw the curtain to obscure her view of Priscilla's bureau, and the infamous "parrot picture" that she still claims is hers.

"Why can't they put up a partition so I can't see that side of the room if those aren't my things?"

"Because the nurses and CNAs need a clear path through the room, Mom."

"What nurses? What are CNAs?"

"You're in a nursing home for physical therapy, and the nurses and assistants are helping take care of you while your hip heals."

"Well, I just don't like it here. In fact, I hate it. I hate seeing those things"—she waves her hand at her roommate's bureau—"and having that woman [her roommate] over there."

"Well, Mom, at least Priscilla is up and out of the room most of the time during the day. I see her out in the hall in her wheelchair every time I'm here. You've really got the room to yourself most of the time. Besides, why don't you get out more? You know they have entertainment downstairs in the lobby. I think it's 'Old Tunes' today—music from the '40s that you used to dance to. Wanna go downstairs?"

"No, I'm not in the mood. I just want to sit here and drink my wine."

The next day, the sitter called me to say that she got Mom downstairs to listen to some people singing Gospel music and that Mom was singing along and clapping her hands. She said that afterwards Mom was "mingling" with everyone, smiling and talking like she'd known them forever. And just a few days earlier she had created a scene in the dining room, saying she didn't know anyone and hated the food.

The sitter said Mom ate a little more on Saturday, and seemed to be in better spirits. I told her where the wine was stashed and asked if she would pour Mom a cup later in the afternoon, and she just laughed and said she'd be happy to. (It's not the same sitter who was reading the Bible to Mom a few days earlier. I have to pick and choose which ones to call on for various tasks.)

Before leaving town I met with Mom's "team" at Manhattan: the director of social services, nurse supervisor, physical therapist, occupational therapist, and speech therapist. The physical therapist thinks Mom needs to stay here 6-8 weeks, rather than the 3-4 weeks I was initially told. And I found out from the nurse that Mom wasn't on any pain meds. So they expect an 80-year-old with

Alzheimer's to do painful physical therapy a week after surgery for a broken hip? The nurse agreed to ask the doctor for something she could take in a small dose to help her do the therapy. The goal, of course, is to have her walking, even with a walker, and able to get in and out of bed unassisted, so she can return to Ridgeland Pointe. My fear is that she won't improve enough and will be in a nursing home the rest of her life. I know that day might be coming, but I just hope it's not soon.

I had dinner tonight with a group of friends, most of whom have (or have had) parents or relatives in nursing homes. And while the humorous stories that people shared diminished my anxiety over Mother's situation a little bit, it's a delicate peace. The trick is not to picture her in her bed in the nursing home when I crawl into my own bed tonight. That image has haunted my sleep for many nights these past few weeks. But maybe embracing her suffering is part of what it means to be my mother's keeper. I wonder how she handled my grandmother's suffering. I wish I had asked her back in 1986.

If Mama Ain't Happy
Saturday, November 8, 2008

Just before I left Jackson to return to Memphis today, I drove through the parking lot at Maywood Mart Shopping Center, to get a latte at Starbucks for the drive. Strolling slowly past Le Nails and the liquor store and grocery store where Mom used to shop, I stop and watch two older ladies slowly unloading their groceries into their cars. They look to be about Mom's age and well-kept, their grey hair obviously maintained weekly at the beauty parlor. One of them looks familiar. She could easily be someone from Mom's church, luncheon club, or an old neighbor. What struck me was this—what's the difference between them and Mom? How is it they are still living independent lives, out in their cars on this beautiful, colorful November day, free to select the food they will go home and prepare in their kitchens, for themselves, and perhaps even their husbands?

The contrast is stark. Leaving the nursing home where Mom is in rehab for a broken hip, I could barely walk through the halls without running into dozens of elderly folks blocking the crowded space around the nurses' station. Many of them are "trapped" in their wheelchairs with trays that prevent them from falling out. Some of them smile or return my greeting as I pass by, but others stare into space or don't even lift their heads from their trays. Ninety-nine percent of them are Black, which isn't an issue for me, just a demographic that plays into the scenario for Mom. Mom doesn't like to leave her room.

Later I visit another nursing home, looking for a long-term care facility for Mom in case she's not able to return to assisted living. This second facility, Lakeland Nursing and Rehab, is the one where my grandmother lived out the last of her years. Another sharp contrast at this nursing home: there were very few residents in wheelchairs in the halls. Instead most of them were gathered in the social room listening to a woman giving an inspirational talk. I paused and watched and listened, and remembered how my father and others from his church led the singing and gave the devotional every Friday for years in this same room, when my grandmother lived at this nursing home.

As I tour the home, it is obvious that the residents are from a different social bracket than at the facility where Mom is currently rehabbing. Most of them are probably parents of my peers, and the residents, their rooms, and the entire facility have a feeling of attentive care, and, yes, money. (But they do accept Medicaid, I was surprised to learn.)

There's a waiting list for this facility, and I won't know for a few more weeks whether or not Mom will improve enough, mentally, to return to Ridgeland Pointe. She can stay where she is indefinitely, but I keep asking myself if I would want to be there, and how much the place itself is responsible for her unhappiness.

Yes, she's very unhappy now. But her Alzheimer's has been exacerbated by everything she's been through this past month—especially the anesthesia for surgery, a week in the hospital, and now three weeks in another unfamiliar facility. And she really hates having sitters with her all the time, often telling them "I don't need you, you can leave now." But without them, the nursing home would probably have to put Mom in restraints, because she can't remember not to get up and try to walk on her broken hip.

On Friday I went with her for her follow-up visit at the orthopedic clinic. I thought we were going to see the physician who did her surgery, but it turned out our appointment was with his nurse practitioner. We sat in the waiting room for over an hour, of course, and Mom asked me over and over why we were there, and I changed my answers up a bit from time to time, just to keep myself entertained. Sometimes I would say, "The doctor who operated on your hip is going to examine you and see how well it's healing," and other times, "They're going to x-ray your hip and see if you can walk soon."

Throughout this time she complained that her hip hurt and asked why her chair was different from mine, which she was sure was more comfortable.

"You're in a wheelchair, Mom, and besides, this waiting room chair really isn't very comfortable either."

"Why am I in a wheelchair?"

"Because you broke your hip, and you can't put weight on it yet."

Imagine this conversation times ten, at least.

And later Mom asked, "I've forgotten what's wrong with you? Are you sick? Why did I bring you here today?"

Finally we're back in the exam room, waiting for another 15-20 minutes, and Mom begins to say she has to use the bathroom. So I go out in the hall and tell the nurse that Mom is in a diaper, but we're hoping she'll be getting weight-bearing status today so she can use the toilet, and she's been constipated and she really, *really* needs to go, so can someone help her to the toilet?

The nurse says she'll call someone, a "cast technician," so we wait.

The only cast technician around is a male, and he's not allowed to help her to the toilet, so the nurse says to tell Mom to use her diaper and they'll give her a dry one.

Mom says she'll just wait.

Finally they take her across the hall to x-ray and I hear her cry out with pain getting on and off the table. When she returns, we wait again.

Finally the nurse practitioner comes in the room and says, "Why are there still staples in your mother's hip?"

"My name is Susan Cushman, and this is my mother, Effie Johnson. And you are—?"

"Oh, I'm sorry, I'm Betty Bones." (Not her real name.) "We sent your mom home from the hospital with instructions for the nurse at the nursing home to remove the staples from her hip after two weeks. Why weren't they removed?"

"This is the first I've heard, since I'm only the daughter and not an employee of the nursing home."

"Oh, well, we'll get someone to remove them now."

And then she turned to Mom and began to explain how the hip was healing fairly well, but not completely yet, and she needed two more weeks until she could walk on it, but for the next two weeks the physical therapists could start her on gait training or something like that. She used lots of technical medical terms and Mom looked at her like she was speaking Greek. Finally I whispered, "She has Alzheimer's. Can you speak slowly and use more simple terms?"

This slowed her down a bit, and I explained how frustrated (and constipated) Mom was, having been in a diaper for a month now, and could she now use a walker and a toilet? The nurse practitioner said she could if someone helped her, or if she understood that she can't put any weight on her right foot yet. I said we've got sitters 24/7 for that purpose, and she said great, tell them Mom can do that. And I said please write this down for me to take to the nursing home, because the nurses and aides aren't allowed to do anything without the physical therapists' orders, and she said she would.

After they removed the staples, we waited (again) for the nurse to return with instructions, and again Mom asked to use the bathroom.

I went back into the hall and asked the nurse practitioner if someone could help me get Mom to a toilet. She looked at me sadly and said, "I know this sounds mean, but there just aren't enough people here to help her do that right now. We're short-staffed. She'll have to use the diaper."

I looked up and down the hall and counted 5-7 people in uniforms, some standing around, others going in and out of rooms. Then I returned to the exam room and told Mom we were leaving soon, could she wait? And she said she could. I've never felt so helpless, and I fought back tears and tried to keep up a cheerful front for Mom's sake.

We waited another ten minutes, so finally I took Mom (in her wheelchair) out to the front door where the shuttle from the nursing home was picking her up, telling the nurse that I would return for the paperwork.

After putting Mom on the shuttle, I found the nurse, who handed me the instructions to take back to the nursing home. I read over them to be sure they were explicit, and yes, they included the request for a bedside toilet and a walker, and for the physical therapists to begin gait training activities, etc. But at the bottom of the sheet there were three questions, and when I read them and the boxes they had checked (yes or no) I just shook my head and took the sheet back inside to the nurse.

"Why did you say 'no' to the question that says, 'Is patient in need of social/vocational adjustment services?' Mom is receiving physical, occupational and speech therapy at the rehab center because of her dementia and her broken hip. This will tell them to discontinue the OT and cognitive therapy."

The nurse nodded and offered to change it.

"Oh, and also the second question, which says 'Is patient aware of diagnosis/prognosis?'... you checked 'yes,' but she's obviously not aware of anything—she doesn't even remember that she broke her hip. Can you change this one, too?"

The nurse nodded again and took the form back to the computer and returned with a corrected sheet in a few minutes. I left and drove to the nursing home, where Mom was already upstairs in her room picking at her late dinner while her sitter, who had accompanied her in the van, was finishing her own hamburger.

Mom asked the sitter to leave, and then told me (again) how unhappy she is having someone in the room with her all the time. She thinks they are "going through her stuff" when they're just helping her. (Yes, I've checked, and nothing is missing.) "I'm just really unhappy," Mom finally says. This is the most clarity she's shown about her emotions and it crashes through the emotional wall I'm trying to build in order to be able to help her.

"I know, Mom, and I wish I could make everything perfect, but I can't. I'm doing the best I can." I try to fight back the tears, but

I'm so exhausted I let a few fall. "Just like you did for Mamaw, when you had to move her into the nursing home."

"Who is Mamaw?"

"You know what, Mom? I'm going to your apartment to get a few more of your things. I'll be back in about an hour, okay?"

"My apartment? Isn't this my apartment?"

"No, Mom, this is your room in the nursing home where you're staying until your hip gets well and you can walk again." I get back out the pictures of her apartment and ask the sitter to look at them with Mom again while I'm gone.

As I leave the room I hear Mom tell the sitter, "You can leave, too. I don't need anything right now."

I went downstairs and met with the director of social services, and told them about the staples that weren't removed and the orders for a walker and a bedside toilet, and she said it would be Monday before they could get the walker and toilet, which means she has to wait three more days. I consider going to a medical supply house and just buying them myself, but I realize that they probably can't get the "orders" to the nurses and aides to allow this change before Monday anyway, so I'll wait and let Medicare pay for them.

So I'm a bit of a basket case, trying to learn not to let my mother's physical, emotional or mental state control mine. (If Mama ain't happy....) And trying to remember to be thankful for the good times, like Thursday afternoon, when Mother's old neighbors, Donna, Sis and Ed, visited her at the nursing home. Donna Burt and Sis and Ed Kemp lived across the street from my parents for about fifteen years. When my father was dying with cancer, Ed used to drive him to the men's prayer breakfasts at the church, and later just came to sit with him so Mom could run errands. He's about 85 now.

When her visitors first arrived, I'm sure she didn't know them, but after a while she seemed to. Or at least she seemed happy.

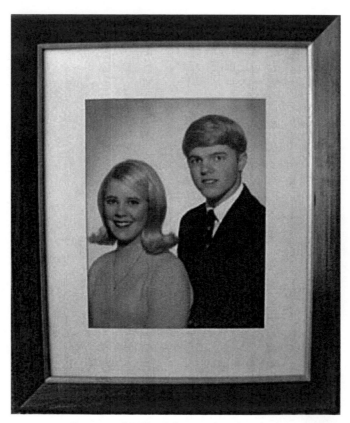

Susan and Mike Johnson (my brother)
1968

The Purse
Friday, November 14, 2008

It's been a difficult month for my eighty-year-old mother. If you've been following my blog, you know she fell and broke her hip, spent a week in the hospital, spent a month in rehab, and yesterday I moved her to Lakeland Nursing and Rehabilitation. I haven't made the final decision that this will be long-term, but I think the chances that her mental status will improve enough for her to return to assisted living are slim.

Not that it's a given, when you break your hip. I visited with a lady who lives in Mom's assisted living facility yesterday who also fell and broke her hip. After three weeks of rehab, she returned to assisted living, with the only change being she uses a walker for support. I asked her where she did her rehab, and she said Lakeland, the nursing and rehab center that I finally got Mom into yesterday. They didn't have any beds available a month ago when Mom was leaving the hospital. I cringed to think that she might be walking by now if she had been in this facility sooner, but what can you do?

The move itself was traumatic, with Mom arguing that I didn't ask her if she wanted to go there, that I only came to town every few months to make decisions for her and then *whoosh* I was gone again. (Not true, of course, but she's lost all sense of time.)

"Mom, I offered for you to live in Memphis, with us, so I could see you more often, but you refused. You said you wanted to stay in Jackson, remember?"

"You would say that!" She was almost in tears now, and Sondra from Comfort Sitters tried to distract her with finishing up dressing her for the move while I packed everything from her drawers and closet, and took all the posters and cards and pictures off the walls. The TV had to be unhooked (and a third appointment made for Comcast to hook her up again) and everything loaded in my car.

We were almost ready when Mom asked, "Where is my purse?"

"It's at my house, Mom, I took it home when you went to the hospital, to keep it safe."

"Well, I need it back now. I can't go anywhere without my purse! What if I need a Kleenex?"

"Here, put some in the pockets of your sweater, sweetie," Sondra offered.

Mom swatted her away. "What about my wallet?"

"It's safe in your purse at my house for a while, Mom."

This brought tears—a rare expression of emotion for Mom. The purse represented independence, and Mom saw for the first time that she had lost her connection with the plastic cards in that wallet. I just couldn't risk her losing them or having them stolen, so I made copies of her Social Security and insurance cards for each facility and kept the originals with me, along with her debit card for the bank account in which I keep a small amount of spending money for her. I check it online, and she hadn't used that card for three months. She rarely goes to the drug store or other errands on the shuttle, and I'm not sure she knows how to use the debit card anymore.

"Mom, you're going to have to trust me about this, I love you, and you need to go to a place where they can help you get your hip healed so you can walk again." I tried to hug her and smooth her hair, but she slapped my hand away.

"Quit touching my hair!" This was a level of anger I hadn't seen in many years. I can't imagine how it must feel to have no control over decisions like these. The responsibility I felt was overwhelming.

As I pushed her down the hall to the elevator, she held a small pillow in her lap, a poor substitute for her purse, but something to hold onto, nonetheless. I'm thinking I need to put a few non-valuable items in her purse and bring it back to her on my next visit. Its presence could be comforting. Or, it could make her anxious about why the wallet is missing.

There's good news and bad news about her arrival at Lakeland Nursing and Rehabilitation Thursday morning. The good news is that it's a lovely facility. It's the one where my grandmother lived in 1986. The cathedral windows in the lobby give a view to the tall pines outside on the front, and there's a lovely enclosed courtyard in the middle.

Once we got Mom settled in her room, hanging pictures on the walls and along the windows, it began to feel homier. But she kept asking when we were going home. It wasn't sinking in that this was where she was staying.

I miss Sondra (our favorite sitter—we both cried when we said goodbye on her last day). She could always find a way to distract Mom when she was upset. She's from South Africa and spoke with a lovely accent and called mother "Lovie."

Near the end of an exhausting day, a surprise visit cheered us up. Derwood Boyles, my father's childhood friend and roommate at Mississippi State (in the 1940s), came by to see Mom and brought flowers.

Derwood has been a community leader in Jackson for many years. He is a very kind and spiritual man. At one point when Mom said she didn't feel like she was worth much at her age, he said, "Well Moses was about 80 when God used him to do mighty things. But he had to have some help, holding up that staff. We all need help from time to time."

The picture above Mom's bed is of my brother, Mike, and me, when we were 17 and 18. It was a surprise gift to our parents on their 20th wedding anniversary, December 27, 1968. They would be celebrating their 60th next month. I reminded Derwood that Mom and Dad had the habit of saying, "This is the Day the Lord has made," and the other person answering, "Let us rejoice and be glad in it!" every morning, and that my husband and I started doing that when Daddy died. Derwood teared up and said, "Regina [his wife] and I do the same thing—we also learned that from Bill and Effie."

Around sunset Mom and I were sitting in the lobby, enjoying the view, when she looked at her watch and said, "It's getting late.

We need to get going if we're going to get home before dark. What are we doing about supper?"

"You'll have supper in the dining room here tonight, Mom." I pointed behind us, around the corner towards the dining room.

"Do I need money? Where's my purse?"

"It's already paid for, Mom. All of your meals are paid for here. Just relax and enjoy them."

She's lost ten pounds in the month since she broke her hip. And she's picking at her food more and more, no longer enjoying many foods that have been favorites most of her life—like grits—and "forgetting" that she's hungry. Dementia does that. The staff will be alert to try to keep her nourished and hydrated, but they can't force her to eat.

She is allowed to have a glass of wine with dinner, once the doctor "prescribes" it and I provide the ongoing supply for her. I think I want to put that in my will—that whoever is taking care of me when I can no longer make choices for myself will be sure I get a glass of wine every night! It's nice to know Mom's evening cocktail will be served with dinner.

Purses optional.

I'll be heading back to Jackson next Wednesday to take Mom for another checkup with the surgeon. Evidently her hip is healing more slowly than he had hoped, for some reason. The physical therapist at Lakeland spoke with him on the phone today, to clarify Mom's rehab orders. In fact, within an hour of my returning home to Memphis this afternoon, I had received phone calls from four different people at Lakeland, asking for more information about Mom's "social history" and updating me on her progress. The head of social services even gave me her email and says she checks it frequently. The two hundred miles between Jackson and Memphis just shrank considerably. I am so thankful for the good people at Lakeland, whether or not it's Mom's last stop this side of heaven.

Long Distance Caregiving
Wednesday, November 19, 2008

When I moved my mother from one nursing home to another a week ago, more than one person asked me why I didn't move her to Memphis, where I live.

"Wouldn't it be easier for you to take care of her?"

"Well, yeah, but I promised her I would let her stay in Jackson. When we bought a house with a mother-in-law suite just for her, she refused to move in with us—that was three years ago. And she's been really happy in assisted living in Jackson."

"But if she's in a nursing home and her Alzheimer's is worse now, does she really know what city she's in?"

"Maybe not. But her city still knows she's there."

See, Mom has lived in Jackson, Mississippi, for 60 years. She and my dad were among the founding members of Covenant Presbyterian Church back in around 1959, and people from Covenant still visit her—whether she's in assisted living or a nursing home. And even people she no longer recognizes (a quickly growing number) elicit a smile when they remind her of their connection in the past. My peers who live in Jackson and visit their parents at the nursing home speak to her and say they are friends of Susan's, and that means a lot. Sometimes they let me know they've visited her and tell me how she's doing. And I really like the people at the nursing home.

I'm not saying I won't consider moving her to Memphis in the future, but for now, I'm leaving her in Jackson with "her people."

But today was one of those days that challenged my decision. I took Mom back to the orthopedic surgeon who put pins in her fractured hip on October 7, and now the bones have shifted and he's going to do a partial hip replacement... next Tuesday. Two days before Thanksgiving. The good news is she could be up and walking soon afterwards. And yes, I wish they had done the partial hip to begin with, but I'm trying to let go of things in the past I can't fix! Evidently, 85% of non-displaced fractures like Mom's heal with the pins, but I'm not sure the surgeon understood he was operating on a woman with Alzheimer's who could not remember not to put any weight on her foot for a month. She probably displaced the fracture accidentally since then, although I hired 24/7 sitters for a month to try and prevent that. She just can't remember her hip is broken, even for five minutes. So, I went through the mental gymnastics: if Mom had been living in Memphis when she broke her hip, could I have gone to the hospital with her and told the doctor to do the partial and not the pins? No—I was in Seagrove Beach, Florida, when she broke her hip, and couldn't get to Jackson in time for the surgery, and couldn't have made it back to Memphis for sure. I just can't be totally available every minute of every day.

So, next week I'll be driving to Jackson for the surgery, not from Memphis, but from Fairhope, Alabama, where I'll be at "Southern Writers Reading," from Friday through Monday. Five friends from our Oxford writing group have rented a B&B on the Mobile Bay for the weekend. It should be an awesome weekend… if I can quit worrying about my mother while I'm there.

And then the day after the surgery I'll leave her in the hands of the wonderful "Comfort Keepers" (24/7 sitters) while I return to Memphis to prepare Thanksgiving for my husband and our daughter, who's coming home from UT Knoxville (grad school) for the holiday. Mom will return to the nursing home, probably the day after Thanksgiving, and I'll head back down to see her the following week.

My comfort level made some huge leaps today when I met Mom's physical therapist, Marzelle. Like my favorite sitter from Comfort Keepers, Sondra, Marzelle is from South Africa. I think these are the only two people I've ever met from South Africa, and both ended up as two of my mother's best caregivers. She went with Mom and me to Mom's appointment with the surgeon today, to talk with him firsthand about her therapy when she returns to the nursing home. It made such a difference to have her with us. She is kind and compassionate and personable and everything you'd want someone to be if they are helping your mother learn to walk again. She'll be waiting for Mom's return to the nursing home after the surgery, ready to hold her hand and gently coach her through recovery. Having folks like Marzelle on the job makes it much easier to be a long-distance caregiver.

Their Own Special Utopia
Monday, November 24, 2008

One hundred years ago, in 1908, five hundred "free thinking people" seeking "their own special utopia" established the town of Fairhope, Alabama, on a bluff overlooking the Mobile Bay. It started as a community of artists, writers and craftsmen, and it continues to boast many of those talented folks today.

How fitting that this town now plays host to one of the most eclectic gatherings of those writers every November for the annual "Southern Writers Reading" event.

I've been staring at this computer screen for two hours waiting to be hit with something really brilliant to write about the weekend, but I'm posting from a hotel room in Jackson, Mississippi, having spent the afternoon at the hospital with my mother. She's having a partial hip replacement tomorrow. But she has no idea where she is or why. The contrast is stark—between the creative energy at work during the weekend in Fairhope and the quickly diminishing flicker of light in my mother's mind.

I am terrified of surgical procedures, and could barely sleep the night before my surgery for cervical cancer in 2001. But Mother sleeps in peace tonight, oblivious to what tomorrow brings. Over and over this afternoon, she opened the musical card I brought her that plays "Day by Day" from the musical *Godspell* and is each time amazed anew at the miracle of the music coming from the greeting card. She watches the sun set from her hospital window and asks where she will sleep tonight.

"Right here, in your bed, Mother."

She doesn't question me, other than to ask where I will sleep.

"I'll be right down the street, at the Cabot Lodge, and I'll be back in the morning, before your surgery."

"Surgery?"

"For your broken hip, remember?"

"Oh, it doesn't bother me much. But I'll see you in the morning."

I kiss Mom, then I hug Sondra, our very special sitter, and leave for my hotel room as Mother picks at the chicken and turnip greens and cornbread on her tray. She smiles.

"See you in the morning, Mom." And I drive down the street to my hotel.

By the time I check in and unpack, my magical weekend in Fairhope feels much more than twenty-four hours and two hundred miles away. I look over my notes—names of writers and agents and publishers I met and networked with all weekend, nuggets of brilliance and kindling for the fire that burns in my creative soul.

My camera is full of images from a weekend spent with friends from my writing group and the talented group of artists, musicians and writers who gathered to share their gifts. And my heart is full of gratitude for the amazing hospitality of the good people of Fairhope who opened their homes to us vagabonds for dinners and breakfasts all weekend long.

But tonight I have no strength for writing about the gifts of the weekend or downloading the photos. Maybe tomorrow night. Tonight I will use my dwindling energy to say a prayer for my mother's healing at the hand of the surgeon tomorrow. And for her continued peace in the midst of the growing fog. May she meet God in the cloud as Moses did. May she find her own special utopia.

Stepping Up
Excerpt from post on
Sunday, November 30, 2008

It's a lot to take in. Beth just left to return to grad school in Knoxville, and tomorrow I'll make the familiar drive back down to Jackson to visit my mother in the nursing home, and begin cleaning out her assisted living apartment. She won't be returning to her apartment, since she now needs a higher level of care. It was a wonderful home for her these past two and a half years, and the folks there are sad to be losing her.

My prayer is that her new little world at Lakeland Nursing Home will become a peaceful haven for this part of her journey. And that she'll be up and walking on her "new" hip so she can get around the facility talking to everyone and flashing them that winning smile, even through the clouds that Alzheimer's keeps building around her mind.

Bingo! And Birthdays Lost
Monday, December 1, 2008

I visited my brother's grave today, in Ridgeland, Mississippi. December 1 is Mike's birthday. He would be 59 years old, if he hadn't died of lung cancer in January of 2007.

The big tree near his grave offers shade from the hot Mississippi sun when I visit during the summer.

But today it was cold and cloudy up on that windy hill. The smaller trees lining the cemetery still had some of their orange glow, as if they were holding onto their last bit of life before joining the dark sky in its wintry palette.

Mike's grave is only a few feet away from my father's and my goddaughter Mary Allison's graves. I wish I had taken new silk flowers (live flowers aren't allowed here) but that will have to wait for another visit. Mom used to keep a broom and a bottle of water in her trunk and she would use them to clean my father's tombstone each time she visited. She would sit on the bench under the big tree afterwards and remember their almost fifty years together. December 27 would be their 60th wedding anniversary.

That precious memory is growing dim as quickly as those beautiful leaves are fading. When I visited Mom at the nursing home today, I reminded her that it was Mike's birthday, and she said, "Mike?"

"Yes, Mother, Mike—my brother—your son. He would be 59 today. He died almost two years ago."

She only stared at me. No response at all. This is a new level of loss. Since she wasn't sad, I tried to cheer myself up by decorating her nursing home room with a small Christmas tree and a pine swag for her wall, and I couldn't help but remember Christmases

71

past. While we were in her room Mom kept asking, "How will I know where my room is?"

I wheeled her into the hall and pointed to her door, which had her name on it. "Look, Mom, it's room 322 and it has your name on it."

"Oh, okay. And where will I get those, oh, you know, I take them with water…."

"Your medicines?"

"Yes!"

About then another resident wheeled up next to us and said, "Right here!" And indeed the nurse was giving out meds just then. She came up to Mom and gave her a hug and Mom smiled and laughed. She just seemed to need to know that there was some order, somewhere, if not in her own mind.

When I first arrived today, Mom was in the lobby visiting with two friends from her church. I was so happy to find her with visitors! She's still in a wheelchair, although the physical therapist has her doing a little walking with a walker, but not on her own yet. But she's not complaining of pain, thank God.

Later we went to the dining room to get a cup of coffee and discovered that it was almost time for bingo. We joined a nice man who was sitting alone at one of the tables and I introduced Mom and myself to him. The man was clear-thinking and friendly as Mom struggled to make cohesive conversation. He smiled kindly and winked when Mom couldn't remember how to play bingo and I tried to help her with her card. They've got these cards with little transparent plastic red "windows" that slide over the number, rather than loose pieces that you cover the number with. Mom was fascinated with them and kept covering up random numbers and I had to keep uncovering them so we could see when she did, in fact, have five in a row.

Mom won bingo twice, so she got lots of chocolate candy, which she proceeded to devour more quickly than I can ever remember seeing her enjoy any food. When the young teenage girl who was volunteering at the nursing home brought the box of candy over for Mother to choose one when she won, Mom started getting packages for everyone at our table, not understanding that only the winner got one. So when the girl walked away, Mom began to share her candy with the table, apologizing for the silly rules. Go, Mom!

I Hope You Dance
Excerpt from post on
Friday, December 5, 2008

Mom's physical therapist at the nursing home called today. They can't get Mom to cooperate with therapy. She's in a wheelchair and might not ever walk again if she doesn't do the physical therapy. But she doesn't understand, or remember, that her hip is broken, or that she can't walk. So they were asking for my help... for any suggestions.

I said, "She loves to dance. Put on some Benny Goodman and entice her onto the dance floor."

"That might work," the therapist agreed. "What else did she like to do in her past life? Did she garden or sew or paint or—"

"She was in a garden club and a luncheon club, and she painted in college, but we couldn't get her to paint later in life. She sort of pulled out of her social circles when she and Dad started their own business, Phidippides Sports, in 1982. Mom ran the aerobic dancing part of the business. So, you could talk to her about aerobics at Phidippides and maybe that would get her going!"

This therapist was hanging on my every word, looking for something that might work. How can I ever thank her enough? These are good people.

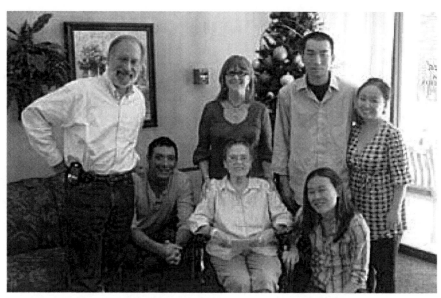

Bill Cushman, Susan Cushman, Jason and See Cushman (standing)
Jonathan Cushman, Effie Johnson, Beth Cushman (seated)
Christmas Holidays, 2008, Lakeland Nursing Home

Somebody's Grandmother
Excerpt from post on
Monday, December 29, 2008

The day after Christmas my family piled into two cars and headed down from Memphis to Jackson to visit Granny Effie. Our caravan included my husband and me, our oldest son, Jon, our second son, Jason, and his wife, See, and our daughter, Beth. Jon would be leaving from there to head back to Savannah, where he is stationed with the Army. Jason and See would return to Memphis with us and then fly home to Denver. Beth would return to the University of Tennessee in Knoxville where she was finishing up graduate school.

I'm not sure if Mom really knew all her grandkids or not, but she loved the visit and seemed to understand that See was new, whether or not her Alzheimer's kept her from getting the concept that Jason was married. Or that they would be providing her with her first great-grandchild next July.

We visited in the lobby of the nursing home, where she opened gifts and enjoyed the comings and goings of other visitors. Jason was unusually quiet, at times on the verge of tears.

"It's just hard for me to see her here."

"I know. Me, too. But it's the best we can do for her right now." I knew Jason was probably thinking similar thoughts to mine when I was angry at my mother for putting her mother in a nursing home.

We posed for group pictures.

I'm always wondering which year will be the last, so each year has its own special meaning. I was so proud of our children for wanting to make the trip, as difficult as it was. I thought about all the times they visited nursing homes in Memphis to sing Christmas carols with their classmates from the elementary and middle school they attended. And how much easier that was because they didn't know any of the people they were singing to. Maybe now they can better understand how much their music meant to those people who were somebody's mother. Somebody's grandmother.

Pushing the Right Buttons
Saturday, January 10, 2009

Mom is almost eighty-one now, and has had a diagnosis of Alzheimer's for several years. After my father died in 1998, I began to visit her more frequently, and eventually began doing her taxes and other bookkeeping. Thankfully, while she was still thinking clearly, she made me Durable Power of Attorney and put my name on her bank account and investment account, so that I could manage everything for her more smoothly. Several people who are just beginning to take care of aging parents have asked me about various aspects of caregiving, and this is one thing I strongly recommend, if the parent(s) are open to it. Especially where Alzheimer's is concerned.

When I moved Mother to an assisted living home in February of 2006, I took her to the bank first and we opened a second joint checking account. I gave her a debit card and a checkbook for this account only, and I put $200 in it, so she could have a little money when the shuttle took her to the drug store or other errands. By watching her account online, I could transfer money from her main account whenever she needed it. All her bills have been coming to me in Memphis (or automatically drafted from her account) for the past three years, which makes the financial end of things fairly simple. If only the physical, mental and emotional aspects were so easy!

I watch her disappear into her own world a little bit more with each visit to her nursing home. Since October, those visits have been almost weekly, but now that she's settling in, I'm comfortable with making the trip every two to three weeks. My most recent visit was yesterday.

First I called Marzelle, Mom's physical therapist, to let her know I was coming, so she wouldn't schedule Mom's PT during my visit. Marzelle was glad I called, because she wanted to tell me a story:

"Yesterday your mom got up on the wrong side of the bed. She was grumpy and wouldn't cooperate with me at all, and even snapped at me angrily. Another resident who was in the physical therapy room at the same time noticed her behavior, and later I saw them talking in the hallway, their wheelchairs side by side.

"The next time I ran into your mom, she stopped me and said, 'Oh, I want to apologize for being so mean to you earlier. You are always so nice to me, and I don't know why I was so mean. Please forgive me.'

"I was flabbergasted. She seemed so lucid, to remember her behavior, and to genuinely ask forgiveness. Of course I told her I didn't take it personally, I knew she was having a difficult time. And then she went back to being her usual cheerful self. She's wheeling up and down the halls all the time now, smiling at everyone, and going into people's rooms to talk with them."

What amazed me about this is that I don't ever remember Mom acknowledging her own meanness, and there was plenty of it over the years. She's always related on a superficial level, at least with me. She's always given the appearance of being in control of her emotions. When I told a friend about this, she said maybe it's too painful for my mother to be in touch with her feelings, so she's always hidden behind a superficial personality. I think there's some truth to that. When I was growing up, she was always either extremely cheerful or bitingly critical, nothing in between. (I think I have those same tendencies, and have to work at being authentic.) Her father was overly strict, and I even suspect he might have abused her, as he did me, when I was very young. The sins of the fathers.

Anyway, I found Mom in the hall near her room and we went into her room to visit. I took her some cookies from McAlister's Deli, her favorite, which she gobbled up, and a pretty "suncatcher," which I attached to her window. She pointed to things in her room, like the calendar on the wall, and said, "I've been writing down some dates and trying to get things in order." Then she pointed to a stack of newspapers on her tray and said,

"And I've been doing some reading, you know—to understand the directions about where to go and when and all that."

After a few minutes, Marzelle found us and asked Mom if she wanted to show me how much progress she's making with her walking. She brought the walker into the room and helped Mom to her feet. Out in the hall, she took a few steps and then pushed the walker away and said, "Someone else can have a turn now." She started to walk on her own (which her hip can't sustain yet) and Marzelle caught her and put her hands back on the walker.

"I can walk whenever I want to!" Mom exclaimed. She still has no idea that she broke her hip or needs help.

Later we meet up with "Henry" (not his real name), the fifty-something man who is in the nursing home because of a stroke. His mind is clear and he rides around in a motorized wheelchair, but his speech is difficult to understand.

"My computer is broken," I finally understand him to say, as he and Mom and I are visiting in the hall near the door to his room, which is full of books, a TV, desk, computer and lots of photos of him with friends. It saddens me that he's stuck in a nursing home, his mind trapped in a body that won't work. I always try to visit with Henry each time I'm there.

Mom starts waving her hands around in the air, and then points with her index finger as though she's pushing an imaginary keyboard and says, "Well, when you get old like us, you just have to keep pushing all the buttons until one works." Henry and I exchange looks, smile, and then break out laughing. Sometimes you just have to laugh.

Later we go out onto the patio (it's 70 degrees on January 9!) where it's sunny and the birds are at the feeders and there's a nice breeze. Mom begins to point to the doors to each wing that opens onto the patio—the dining room, the physical therapy room, and the doors to the main lobby.

"Those doors are probably locked, which is fine with me. I don't want to buy anything today."

"What do you buy in there, Mom?"

"Oh, sometimes there's coffee, but they're still working on that part." And then she looks at her hands and points to her fingernails and adds, "And I've been trying to get them all even but I don't want to paint them right now so I keep telling them just to keep them even." Her nails are a nice length, obviously clipped and filed recently. Her hair is shoulder-length, for the first time in about fifty years. The beautician at the nursing home will cut and perm Mom's hair, if she will let her.

"Your hair looks pretty, Mom. Have you decided not to get it cut anymore?"

"Oh, I just haven't been in the mood."

About then the director of social services and another woman who works in the front office come out onto the patio for a smoke. They are sitting on a bench near the back side of the patio, and Mom starts "paddling" (making the wheelchair go with her feet) towards them, so I follow along beside her.

"Hi!" Mom says.

"Hi, Miss Effie," they reply.

"This is my daughter." Of course they already know me, since I've been there almost weekly for the past three months. "She doesn't come to see me very often." My inner child wants to say, "Oh, yes I do, Mom! I'm a Good Daughter!" But I just smile and we keep moving.

A group of residents has gathered around a nearby table as the recreational director brings in a short basketball goal and ball and starts getting some of them to play.

"Do you want to go and visit with them, Mom?" I ask.

"Oh, no. They're always here. Let's go back inside."

We enter the lobby and Mom says, "Let's go down this way." So I go along with her to the transitional care unit, where the physical therapy room is. On the way down the hall she looks into every room, waving and speaking to everyone. In one room a woman about my age is standing beside her mother's bed and Mom wheels into the doorway so I follow. The woman has something wrong with her legs and can't walk, but her mind is clear, so I introduce Mom and me and she and her daughter do the same. Then the woman asks, "How long have you been here?"

Mom stares blankly, so I answer for her. "Mom came here on November 15, after two hip surgeries. Before that, she lived at Ridgeland Pointe Assisted Living for about three years."

With that answer, Mom touches my arm and says, "But I've been knowing *her* all her life."

We visit a few minutes, then head up to the front lobby, where there's a nice view of the park next door with the huge pine trees. Mom wheels up beside a couch, so I sit on the couch, and she hands me a copy of a glossy home decorating magazine and says, "Here, I think you might enjoy this. If you're ready for bed, you can just take it with you to your room. Are you tired?"

"No, Mom, I'm fine. I just want to visit with you for a while."

"Well, I need to go down the hall and check on something. You just rest here with your magazine and I'll see you later." With that she turned and headed away from me, down the hall towards her room. I got up and watched her, as she stopped to talk with people along the way, and looked into the dining room, where coffee and donuts would be served at 3 p.m. I realized then that she had just brought me into her new world. I had become another resident there. One who might enjoy a magazine, or might need a nap. My eyes filled with tears, and I realized that it might not be long before she wouldn't know me at all when I arrive for a visit. So I hurry after her and give her a hug and kiss and say, "Bye, Mom. I've got to go now. I'll be back soon!"

In the past, whenever I would be leaving her, she would protest a bit, saying, "Oh, do you have to go already?" But this time, she just waved her hand in the air and said, "I'll see you in a little while. I've got to take care of something else right now." And there she was, off to try and figure out how to push the right buttons.

Reality Bites: Granny Effie and "Henry"
Saturday, January 24, 2009

Every time I visit my mother in the nursing home, I take time to visit with the facility's youngest resident, "Henry," whom I've mentioned before. Sadly, Henry is only 55 years old. He appears to have had a stroke, but it could be something else. He uses an electric wheelchair, and his speech is difficult to understand, but his mind is alert.

The last time I was there, Henry said he was having trouble with his remote control and would I come look at it. I went to his room, just down the hall from Mom's, and there he had a computer, lots of books, a television, and shelves of photographs of himself with friends—which must have been taken before whatever tragic event landed him in the nursing home. Radiant smiles are on all the photographs, and the other people in the pictures are attractive, and appear to be active members of society.

So when I drove down to see Mom on Friday, sure enough Henry found us visiting in the front lobby and wheeled over to visit with us. My dear friend Sissy Yerger had met me for lunch and had gone with me to visit Mom. When I introduced Henry to Sissy, Henry said, "Are you related to Wirt Yerger?"

"Yes, he's a distant cousin of my husband," Sissy replied.

Now usually when I'm visiting with Henry, it's hard to include Mom in the conversation for two reasons—for one thing, she can't understand what he's saying very well due to his speech impairment, and she can't follow the conversation or remember most of the people we're talking about. So, it's always a balancing act, to be sure Henry doesn't "take over" the time and attention I'm trying to give to Mom, but to also be sure I'm spending time with him, as he's bound to be starved for company with folks his/our age.

"He was in the insurance business, wasn't he?" Henry continues, talking about Wirt Yerger.

"Yes," I interject, "and so was my father, Bill Johnson."

I look at Mom, trying to draw her into the conversation, and she smiles a faraway smile but nods, so I feel that I'm succeeding.

"How long was your father in the insurance business?" Henry asks me, and then he looks at Mother.

"Hmmmm." I have to think about this. "For about thirty years, I think. And when he retired from that, he and Mother opened Bill Johnson's Phidippides Sports. Dad was a marathon runner, and Mom helped manage the store and organize the aerobic dance business."

Mom is smiling and nodding, but not jumping into the conversation as I hoped she might. With each visit I realize I've lost more of her, fearing each time that she won't know me. But she surprised me with what she said next:

"He was with the F.W. Williams State Agency of U.S.F.&G. Insurance Company."

The words rolled off her tongue as though she said them several times a day. Dad retired from U.S.F.&G. in 1982—27 years ago—and yet this information was such a big part of her memory that it's not lost yet. Interesting how the brain works. She couldn't remember if she had lunch or not, did physical therapy that day or not, but she could repeat this rather complex name of the company my father worked for so long ago.

As we walked up and down the halls a few times, as we do each time I visit—Mom "pedaling" along with her feet in her wheelchair, me at her side—we ran into Mia, the nurse in charge of her wing. "Your mother is fitting in here perfectly," were Mia's words this time, which brought me great comfort.

A few minutes later one of the aides stopped and chatted with us—she and Mom exchanged a few light-hearted teasing comments to each other—and then the aide said to me, "Miss Effie tries to pretend that she's a bad girl, but we know better."

Interesting comment. Later Mom told me that she "got into a row" with someone that morning (probably the physical therapist) who wanted her to do something she didn't want to do, and that later someone else "fussed at her" for not eating her lunch. I found her lunch tray in her room, so she must not have been in the mood to go to the dining room that day. I picked up the aluminum cover off her plate to see the stale French fries and sandwich, mostly untouched.

But she seems to have put back on some of the weight she's lost since she broke her hip 3 ½ months ago, so I'm not worried about her nutrition. And each time I visit I pick up two giant cookies from McAlister's Deli and she inhales them as we visit, so she hasn't forgotten how to eat!

This time, when Sissy and I were leaving, Mom came up to the front lobby to see us out, and it saddened me to see her watching us go through the doors to my car. She seemed more aware that someone dear had just left her world, whereas last time I left, she dismissed me as if I was another resident with a room down the hall. As much as I hate Alzheimer's and what it does to the mind, there are times when it seems to cushion the difficult truths. The truths about all that she has lost—her life partner of almost fifty years, her independence, her physical strength, and significant portions of her mind.

And I look at Henry, trapped in a facility for old people because of his physical limitations, and I wonder whose truth is the most difficult. Yeah, reality bites.

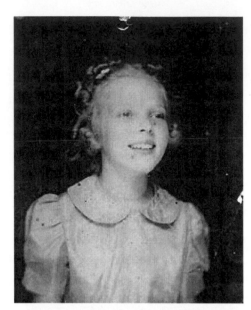

Effie Watkins (1939 and circa 1940)

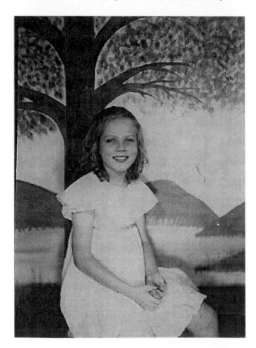

Effie at Eighty-One
Friday, February 20, 2009

Today is my mother's birthday. She's eighty-one.

The first picture on the previous page is Mom when she was eleven years old, in 1939. And this second picture doesn't have a date on back, but she appears to be about the same age, maybe twelve. I love these pictures of her when she was a little girl. And yes, I see some of myself in her then. And also now.

In my post about her this time last year, when she turned eighty, she was still in an assisted living home—still clinging to the last bits of independence that she could grasp. But she was happy in her ever-shrinking world, and I hoped against hope that it would last for a few more years.

And then the inevitable happened. In October she fell and broke her hip, and you know the rest of the story.

I went to visit Mom on Tuesday this week, rather than today, her actual birthday. She has no idea what day it is, but she still lights up when she sees my face. Each time I drive down to Jackson, I wonder if that will be the visit when it happens—when she doesn't know who I am.

First I stopped at Beemon's Drugs at Maywood Mart, in my old neighborhood. Beemon's is one of those old-fashioned drug stores that carry lots of cute gifts and knickknacks—the perfect place to gather goodies for Mom's birthday. Into the gift bag went:

- *Good Housekeeping* magazine (because the pictures are pretty and colorful, and she loves that, even though she no longer reads the articles).
- M&Ms.
- Chewing gum.
- A stained-glass cross to hang on her window.
- Lipstick and blush-on.

- A new comb, brush, and barrettes (she's not letting the beautician at the nursing home cut or perm her hair).
- A lavender (her favorite color) plastic makeup bag to put the new goodies in.

Next I went across the parking lot to McAlister's to get two giant cookies—her favorites—and included them in the gift bag.

Off to Lakeland Nursing Home I went, to find Mom not scooching up and down the halls in her wheelchair, as she usually is, but sitting in her room visiting with her new roommate, Mrs. Jackson, who is 86 and in her right mind. I think. The reason I think so is because she was able to tell me all about her son, her previous situation, and then to announce rather matter-of-factly: "This is the end of the line for me."

"What do you mean?" I asked.

"I mean I guess I'll live here until I die." Mom seemed nonplussed, as she piddled around with her birthday card and gifts. We had fun, putting on her new lipstick and blush-on and holding up her new mirror so she could see how pretty she looks. (If only my skin would look like hers when I'm 81!)

"We get along pretty well," Mom said, pointing to Mrs. Jackson. "Come on over here and have some of my birthday candy." She waved at Mrs. Jackson, who was stretched out on her bed because her back was hurting.

"No, thank you. I've got plenty of candy from Wal-Mart." She pointed to what looked like a display on a candy aisle at a discount store. "I used to work there," she explained.

I kept asking Mom if she didn't want to go up to the lobby to visit, thinking she would want to get out of her room for a while.

"No, I'm fine here. Just look at those beautiful trees!" She pointed out her window to the huge pines on the city park property next door.

"But I need to go to the bathroom," she said.

"Mom, you have on a diaper, remember? You just go when you need to and the nurses will clean you up."

"But she goes to the bathroom on her own sometimes," Mrs. Jackson interjected.

"Really?" I don't even try to hide my surprise. "Do the nurses know this?"

"I don't know, but she goes in there and gets on the toilet sometimes."

Mia, the head nurse, dropped in shortly after this conversation, so I stepped out into the hall to ask her about it and she said, "Oh, yes. She's figured out how to unhook the alarm so we don't know she's out of her wheelchair. She gets the diaper off and gets herself onto the toilet. Sometimes we have to help her get the diaper back on."

I was flabbergasted. "But what if she falls?"

"If she falls, she falls. We're doing everything we can, short of restraints, which we don't use here at Lakeland. She's doing fine."

Back in Mom's room, Mrs. Jackson was complaining, "The food here is awful."

So I looked at Mom to see if she agreed, but she was off on another planet, stroking the ribbon on her birthday gift.

"And the plastic covers on these beds are so hot I wake up sweating at night. Do you think we could get something more comfortable?"

I looked at Mom and asked, "Mom, is the bed comfortable enough for you?"

"Oh, yes, it's fine." Her eyes had a bit of a glazed-over look, but her smile was full. I considered for a moment a possible blessing of dementia—Mom no longer cares about the taste of the food or the comfort of the bed.

"And I can't seem to get a television in here," Mrs. Jackson continued. Her son lives in town, so I asked:

"Has your son tried to bring one and get it hooked up? You have to call Comcast a few days ahead of time. But you are welcome to watch Mom's TV whenever you want to." I looked at Mom.

"I don't watch it much anymore."

"What about the news? You used to like to watch the news."

"Yes, sometimes." There was a resignation in her voice that was new.

"Well, it's okay if Mrs. Jackson wants to watch it, right?"

"Oh, sure! Anytime she wants to."

"Well, my son will be bringing mine eventually," Mrs. Jackson said. "And he's going to bring me some pictures for the walls like your mother has." Her walls were bare, whereas Mom's were covered with framed photographs, posters, and a bulletin board filled with labeled pictures—the one her granddaughter put together for her when she was still in assisted living. Another bulletin board was covered with cards.

About then Mom started playing with her new makeup, when Mrs. Jackson brought out some liquid foundation makeup from her drawer and offered it to Mom: "This is the wrong shade for me—would you like to try it?"

Mom took it and smiled, and their eyes met, and for a moment it reminded me of two young girls sharing beauty supplies. Mom hasn't worn liquid makeup in years, but she said, "I might like to try it sometime." And she put it in her makeup bag.

When it was time for me to leave, I asked if Mom wanted to go up to the lobby to see me off, but she said, "No, I'll stay here, thank you."

I kissed her goodbye and told her happy birthday again, and as I left her room, I watched her maneuvering her wheelchair around to the far side of her bed and placing her birthday card in the window with her other cards. I stood and watched to see what she would do next, but she didn't move. It was getting close to sunset, and the deep orange sky behind the increasingly dark trunks of the pine trees was something to behold. And mother would rather look at the sunset through the trees than watch the news on TV. Who can blame her?

Not Becoming My Mother
Thursday, April 9, 2009

I've never served on jury duty. The only time I was ever asked to was the exact week that our adopted daughter would be arriving from South Korea, in November of 1985. I panicked when I received the letter from the United States District Court ordering me to appear. Thankfully it only took a quick phone call and a simple explanation of my situation for me to be excused. That was 24 years ago. So when a similar letter arrived in my mailbox earlier this week, I thought, "Okay, I can do this now." But the letter wasn't for me. *It was for my mother.* All her official business mail has been coming to my address since I became her Durable Power of Attorney three years ago. I opened the form and began to fill out the questionnaire.

Do you read, write speak and understand the English language? I bubbled in the "yes" circle, although it's a stretch to say that Mom "understands" much of anything these days. Where would there be a place to explain her situation? Ah… there it was:

Do you have any physical or mental disability that would interfere with or prevent you from serving as a juror? I bubbled in "yes" and turned the form over to the "Remarks" section and briefly explained that Mom is 81 years old, has Alzheimer's, is in a nursing home, confined to a wheelchair since her Alzheimer's prevented her full recovery from a broken hip and two surgeries this past fall.

Then under *Grounds for Requesting Excuse,* one of three "grounds" available was: *All persons over 70 years of age.* It didn't say this would be a given, so I wondered if someone who was still alert, but over 70, would be excused. At any rate, I filled out both pages of the questionnaire and dropped it in the mail yesterday.

The same day my copy of *Preserving Your Memory: The Magazine of Health and Hope* arrived in my mailbox. It's published by the Fisher Center for Alzheimer's Research Foundation. I've shared a couple of copies with friends because I find it helpful—short, pertinent, and easy to read. There's an article in the current issue about a new book by Leeza Gibbons called *Take Your Oxygen First* that's coming out in May, specifically for Alzheimer's caregivers. Since my maternal grandmother also suffered from Alzheimer's disease, as did Leeza's, I'm interested in learning all I can.

All this was on my heart as I drove down to Jackson today for a pre-Easter visit with my Mom at her nursing home. I took her a battery-operated "Bunny Hopper" for a laugh. Although I also took Mom a basket of Easter candy, she still enjoys watching the Bunny Hopper, a year later.

It was a gorgeous day to sit on the patio at the nursing home. The trees were greening up and the flowers were blooming, birds were on the bird feeders. Just lovely. As I commented on how pretty the courtyard area was, Mom said, "Yes, I'm so proud of everyone. We've been doing the work a little at a time. I helped with the flowers." This is the same thing she told me on my last visit. I couldn't help but be glad that she enjoys helping with the flowers, if only in her mind.

A young mother with two little girls came by, giving out Easter candy to the residents. Mom was confused, thinking that she should give some of her candy to the girls instead. I guess it is a reversal of roles that one never quite gets used to. Mom was the ultimate holiday person—making a huge deal out of every celebration.

But when we sat quietly for a while, and I managed not to rush to fill the silences, she would stare off into the sky and there's no telling where she went, as she would say things like, "The numbers are sometimes up, up, up" and her hand would point up, "and then sometimes they are down, down, down." Later I wondered if she'd been watching the news about the economy, because she added, "I heard something about where we need to put our money. Do I need to be doing something about that?"

"No, Mom. I'm taking care of all that for you."

"Oh, thank you, dear. You're such a good daughter." She was more subdued than usual. The nurses had told me they had increased some of her psychotropic meds since my last visit because she had become agitated a good bit.

An hour or so went by with only pleasantries being exchanged. She would ask about family members, whose names she doesn't remember, but her face lit up when I told her (again) that she was going to be a great-grandmother soon. And that her granddaughter, Beth, was going to travel to Europe this summer. At one point an aide that helps Mom with personal hygiene joined us. She told me how Mom cared about how her slacks and blouses matched and sometimes needed ironing. She talked about how pretty Mom's hair and skin were, and how Mom had been enjoying wearing a little makeup recently. (I didn't comment that it was overdone—I think the foundation Mom's roommate gave her is two shades too dark!)

Anyway, the aide was real attentive, and after a while she asked me, "Has your mom always been so sweet? I mean, was she sweet to you when you were growing up?"

This struck me as an odd thing to ask, personal, invasive. But I wondered if she understood that often Alzheimer's changes people's personalities, sometimes even for the better. When Mom wasn't looking, I shook my head. The aide gave an understanding nod and smiled gently.

A few minutes later the "old mom" peeked back out briefly. A young woman who was considerably overweight walked through the courtyard. Mom looked at her, then at me, and puffed her cheeks out with air in imitation of the woman and said, "They shouldn't let the big ones in here—they ruin the beauty of it."

Sigh. So much of my life I felt like that's exactly what I did—ruin the beauty of her world by being overweight. Her barbs about my weight left permanent wounds, leading to eating disorders, depression, and other issues. But today I tried not to let her words sting. They weren't directed at me, but at the generic world of imperfect bodies that have always bothered her.

Driving home to Memphis, I thought about a book I had just read. A short memoir by Ruth Reichl called *Not Becoming My Mother*. I received the book in the mail from the marketing department at Penguin Press—it's actually an advance proof they were giving away on Twitter. Only 112 pages, so I read it in one sitting, and it was refreshing seeing the way another daughter dealt with her mother's issues—in this case late diagnosed bipolar disease, but also repression by an era and a generation that held women back from their potential. Her mother told her, "Once you find out who you are, you will find your beauty. You have to grow into your face." Ruth's mother had been told, as a teenager, that she was ugly, and Ruth felt the same way about herself during her own adolescence. She was determined not to pass this on to her own daughter, and her mother's gift to her was to free her not to become her mother.

I've spent most of my life trying not to become my mother. But today, I'm also embracing my own mother where she is, forgiving the past and trying to be thankful for the present. It's a lot to hold onto all at once, without losing myself in the process.

My Mother's Keeper Part II
Monday, June 22, 2009

I haven't been able to quit thinking about the conversation I had with a mother of young children, the one I posted about last Tuesday. I think it's because I've just spent lots of time on the phone trying to straighten out some of my mother's business affairs—I'm her Durable Power of Attorney—and at the end of the day, it can be just as trying as dealing with teenagers, toddlers and newborns. Only without the joys to be had from those precious teenagers, toddlers and newborns!

Please believe that I'm not writing this to complain, but rather to share some of the ins-and-outs of being a full-time daughter of a parent with Alzheimer's. Okay, right away I can hear some of ya'll thinking, "She's not full-time—her mother doesn't live with her. In fact, she doesn't even live in the same city!" And you would be correct on the second two points, but completely wrong on the first one. There is not a day, and some days not an hour, that goes by in which I don't think/worry about my mother and how she's doing. And between visits (usually every 2-3 weeks) I'm taking care of her business from home. Sometimes it's unbelievably complicated. I'll share a couple of stories.

When I moved Mother into an assisted living home in February of 2006, I spent the next three months cleaning out her house and selling it. (Thank God it was before the current financial recession!) One friend helped me go through everything my parents had collected in their forty-nine years of marriage. Mom was a bit of a hoarder. I threw away over seventy large black trash bags of junk, after giving almost that many bags of things to Goodwill and a local church youth group for a garage sale. The job pretty much consumed my life for all of the spring of 2006. Once we moved her into her assisted living apartment, hung all the pictures on the wall and got her cable TV, telephone, and newspaper subscriptions transferred, she was good to go for a few years. She had put my name on all her financial accounts while she could still think clearly, which helped tremendously. (I can't recommend this strongly enough for anyone caring for elderly parents.) I had already been filing Mom's income taxes for a few years (Dad died in 1998) but when she moved into assisted living I had all her business mail sent to me and I began paying all her bills for her.

Things were actually going along fairly smoothly until last fall when her dementia kicked up a notch and I began to research her options. I could (1) move her "upstairs" to the Alzheimer's unit at the assisted living home, for over $4000/month with no skilled nursing care; (2) move her to a skilled nursing home in Jackson; or (3) move her to a skilled nursing home in Memphis. The decision was hurried up a bit in October when she fell and broke her hip. Following surgery and rehab at one nursing home/rehab center, it became clear her hip wasn't healing, so she had a second surgery and more rehab, but this time I made the decision to move her to Lakeland Nursing and Rehab permanently. In Jackson. That was in November. Just six months ago. But in those six months I have:

- Moved her three times (she moved rooms in the first nursing home);
- Changed her cable TV service three times;
- Changed her permanent mailing address three times;
- Cancelled her phone service once she forgot how to use a phone;
- Labeled all her clothes with a Sharpie pen with her name and room number three times;
- Made about nineteen round trips to Jackson for hospital stays, moves, doctor appointments and visits;
- Changed her monthly draw-down on her Schwab account to cover her increasing expenses and met with financial advisers to learn how to apply for Medicaid when her money runs out;
- Closed one of her two bank accounts;

- Changed her Medicare Part D enrollment from Humana to AARP, at the recommendation of the business manager at the nursing home.

That last one is one of the "stories" I want to share. We enrolled Mom in Humana three years ago, with me being Durable Power of Attorney, so all the paperwork came to me here in Memphis. No problem. But in January when we decided to change her to AARP, I asked for help from a friend of my father's in Jackson, because his daughter handles those kinds of things for his business. She got it set up, and after a while (yes, I should have been paying closer attention and I would have caught it sooner) I realized that the statements were being mailed to Mom at the nursing home. I would find them in her trash can or in a stack of greeting cards, often unopened. So, I called the company to ask them to please mail them to me. Turns out they never got my Durable Power of Attorney back in January, so I had to fax it to them, and call them three times over the next ten days to see if they had attached the DPA to her file yet, before they would even talk with me. Finally I was "in" and I asked them to change her mailing address to my address in Memphis. I was told they couldn't do that because she lived in a different state. After several attempts to talk with a manager, I finally got one, who agreed to put my address as the "secondary" mailing address, which means I would get a copy of all correspondence, but so would Mom. Even when I explained that she has Alzheimer's and doesn't remember how to open an envelope, that the aides have to open her cards for her. Of course I said, "I didn't have this problem with Humana," and they said, "Well, this is a policy of Medicare Part D, so Humana should have been following it." Who makes these rules? Is it expected that everyone will live in the same state as their elderly parents?

And then there's Comcast Cable. When I got the cable guy to set up Mom's TV in her room in the second nursing home, he gave us a "deal" of $34.35/month. He didn't say it was only a promotional offer. But after 2 months the bill went up to

$62.65/month, saying the "promotional offer" had ended. Mom barely even watches TV anymore, but I don't want to take it out of her room just yet because sometimes it's good company for her. So today I called Comcast. I called the 1-800 number on the bill and when I finally got a human voice, she told me that she could only help me if the television was in Memphis. I said, "But why is this 1-800 number on Mom's bill, if she lives in Jackson?" Turns out it's because I live in Memphis, and the bills come to me. So she gave me a 1-877 number to call for Mom's zip code in Jackson. I've tried it several times today and it's always busy. They're "open" 24/7, so maybe I'll try later tonight. But what irony, that living out of state penalizes me with both AARP and Comcast.

I could tell more stories, but I think you get the picture.

Fortunately, the folks at her nursing home are great. I get phone calls from nurses and social workers with updates between my visits, and when they hold their regular "care team meetings," they put me on speakerphone so I can talk with everyone at the meeting—nurse, social worker, dietician, activities director, physical therapist, etc. And when I drive down to visit Mom, I always check in with the nurse and director of social services for the latest updates, or to express any concerns I have. They tell me that people from Mom's church visit her, as well as other folks. That comforts me. If I move Mom to Memphis, she won't know anyone but me. I'm pretty determined to make this long-distance care giving work.

Do I feel any guilt? Oh, yes. Every time I leave the nursing home I remember how angry I was at my own parents when they put my grandmother in the same nursing home in the mid 1980s. I had no idea what was involved in caring for someone with Alzheimer's, and I'm sorry it's too late for me to apologize to Mom for judging her. She just wouldn't understand. And I can't help but imagine myself twenty years down the road needing the same kind of care that Mom is getting now. Would I want my daughter to move me to the town she's living in so I can see her more often? I hope I'll feel the same way Mom did when she refused to move to Memphis three years ago—I hope I'll want my own children to carry on with the lives they are building with their families and careers wherever they live. I also hope that there will be money left in our social security and retirement accounts to cover the level of care that my husband and/or I might need, but that's a discussion for another day.

A Visit From Cousin Sonny
Excerpt from post on
Thursday, August 20, 2009

My mother grew up as an only child in Meridian, Mississippi. Her first cousin, Sonny Hopper, was also an only child, and they lived near each other and were more like brother and sister than cousins. Sonny is a retired Presbyterian minister in Lexington, Kentucky. A few years ago I took Mom on a road trip to visit him, before the Alzheimer's had begun to erase her memories. So it hadn't been too long since she had seen him. And yet.

Yesterday Sonny and his new wife, Barbara, stopped in Jackson to visit Mom at her nursing home, and called me from the lobby to chat and also to let Mom talk with me on their cell phone. I asked Sonny, "Does Mom know who you are?"

"Oh, she says we look familiar," Sonny answered. "And she looks great—seems to be happy here, and that's what matters." Sonny is a good man.

After I chatted with Barbara, she asked if I'd like to speak to Mom. Mother has forgotten how to use a telephone, so she doesn't have one in her room anymore. Barbara held the phone up to Mom's ear and we chatted.

"Hi, Mom! It's Susan."

"Oh, hello, dear. How are you?"

"I'm fine, Mom. Are you enjoying your visit with Sonny and Barbara?"

"Who?"

"Your cousin, Sonny Hopper, and his wife, Barbara, from Meridian."

"Oh, I love the sound of those names."

I can see Mom fingering the air as she speaks, as though she's trying to capture the words and put them with the faces.

"Yes, remember that Sonny was Aunt Bess's son, and you grew up with him in Meridian?"

"Oh, isn't that nice. Yes, that sounds good."

A few minutes later I was back on the phone with Sonny, thanking him for their visit and making sure I had all his contact information. After we hung up, I realized that he's the only living person who knew my mother since she was a child. Oh, how I long to visit with him again and ask lots of questions about her. And her people. My people. (I've got pictures of our visit with Sonny in Lexington a while back, but they're in the attic. Some day they'll be in photo albums. Some day.)

Memories Old and New
Excerpt from post on
Sunday, August 30, 2009

This weekend was full of significant events for me. Starting on Friday, when I drove to Jackson to visit my mother, and also to see some paintings by a high school friend, Kit Fields. It was a routine visit with Mom at Lakeland Nursing Home, where she's been living since November. Every couple of weeks when I drive down, I brace myself for the time when she won't know me. She knew me on Friday, but she couldn't figure out who Grace Cushman was when I showed her pictures of her great-granddaughter. This was the second time I've taken photos of Grace with me. A few weeks ago, she remembered who Jason was (my son, Grace's father) but this time there was a blank look on her face and she kept pointing to him and his wife, See, in the pictures, and asking again who there were. Made my heart so sad.

We were sitting in the dining room, where the movie *A River Runs Through It* was on the big screen TV. Some of the scenes are full of great period clothing, music and dancing from the '30s, and Mom's face lit up when those scenes came on. There was something more familiar to her about the images on the screen than the images in my book of photos of Grace. I guess it's that long-term memory trying to hang on.

Alzheimer's and the Jesus Prayer
Tuesday, October 13, 2009

Three hours into my nine-hour drive down to Seagrove Beach on Monday, I stopped at the nursing home in Jackson to visit my mother. I took her a couple of her blouses, which I had brought home from my last visit to wash and iron. They do her laundry at Lakeland, but they don't iron, and sometimes I just want to see her looking the way she looked most of her life—well groomed. She resists the stylist's efforts to cut and set her hair in the beauty parlor, so it's longer on each visit, and Monday it was pulled back in a ponytail, which actually reminded me of her younger days. One of the aides had applied a little blush and lipstick, and she looked pretty.

She was already in the dining room, waiting for lunch, when I arrived at 11 a.m. She was sitting at a table with three other women, but they weren't talking with each other, and Mother seemed to be staring into the distance, the way old married couples do sometimes when they fall into a comfortable silence. I broke the spell when I touched her shoulder and she burst into a grin.

"Hi, Mom!"

"Well, hi, Susan!" (I breathed an inward sigh of relief. On each visit I wonder if she'll know me.)

We kissed on the lips. She is one of only about five people that I kiss on the lips. Three are girlfriends. One is my husband. Like Julia Roberts said in *Pretty Woman*, it's intimate.

I told her about the blouses, which I had put in the closet (really an armoire) in her room, and she said, "Blouses?" I touched her sleeve and said, "Blouses, Mom, you know, shirts. I washed and ironed a couple for you."

"I haven't been able to find the closet for a long while. Are you sure it's there?"

"It's in your room, Mom. The ladies who help you get dressed know where it is."

"Oh…" Her voice trailed off and she looked away from me, at the woman sitting to her left. "Have you been here long?"

"Forever!" the woman answered.

"But have you met my daughter?"

I made light conversation with the other three women for a few minutes, and then returned my attention to mother. "I brought you some of those cookies you like so much."

"Oh?" Her face brightened. "Where are they?"

"I put them in your room."

"Give them to me now!"

"But Mom, you're about to eat lunch. You can have them for dessert after lunch. Will that be okay?"

"Have what for dessert?"

"The cookies, Mom."

"Oh, are there cookies?" She looked around the table for cookies. I just smiled at the other ladies and re-explained about the cookies to Mom.

But as I was continuing my drive to Seagrove later that afternoon, I thought about how I would feel some day, if I'm in her shoes. Her mother had Alzheimer's, so I'm thinking it wouldn't be unlikely. It's one of those things that keep me up at night sometimes. Is there something I can do that will ease the transition, the pain of loss of a mind? Suddenly it hit me—the Jesus Prayer.

"Lord Jesus Christ, Son of God, have mercy on me, the sinner."

Short version, "Lord have mercy."

I taught it to my father when he was dying with lung cancer.

I watched my friend Urania say it at numerous visits to the cancer clinic, and again during her final days at home before her death two years ago. If it can bring peace during physical illness and impending death, can it also bring peace as Alzheimer's wages war with the brain?

Known as the "prayer of the heart," ascetics have practiced it for centuries, the most skilled amongst them attaining a level of spirituality in which the prayer goes on "on its own" in the heart, almost automatically. Even if the lips aren't saying it aloud.

About fifteen years ago, when I was in a particularly intense period of my life, spiritually, I "practiced" the Jesus Prayer fairly regularly during the day for a number of months, and I found it did bring peace. But then I got lazy and left it behind for a while, picking it back up for a few weeks in 2001 when I was diagnosed with cervical cancer and had to have numerous tests and surgery. I'm a real wimp about pain, and I was afraid of the cancer, so it really helped.

And this afternoon, at times when it was pouring down rain on the highway, so much that I could barely see the cars and trucks in front of me, I found the words returning to my lips, and hopefully, to my heart.

So now I'm thinking if there was ever a case for making the Jesus Prayer a part of my heart forever, it's the thought of Alzheimer's eventually grabbing hold of my brain and gradually shutting it down, trying to steal my soul in the process.

I'm penning this at 11 p.m. on my first night here, alone in a beach house, waiting for four friends and my husband to join me, two on Tuesday, two more on Wednesday, and hubby on Thursday. Even with the French doors to the deck closed, I can hear the waves. The rhythm of the ebb and flow of the tide is a perfect accompaniment:

Lord Jesus Christ... Son of God... have mercy on me... a sinner.

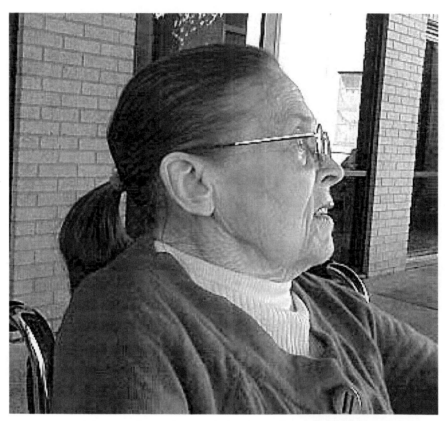

Mom on the patio at Lakeland Nursing Home, 2009

An Unexpected Gift
Tuesday, November 17, 2009

Yesterday was my bi-monthly visit with my mother at Lakeland Nursing Home. If you're new to my blog, Mom is 81 and has Alzheimer's.

As I drove down to visit her, I received a phone call from a dear friend in Memphis. Her mother had fallen and was in the hospital. Another friend's mother had also fallen, a few days ago, and is now staying with her daughter and family as they decide if she can return to her home, assisted living, or other options. And yet a third friend emailed me with news of her father's recent diagnosis with cancer. This business of getting old is complicated, I think, by two things in particular, and probably a whole slew of things in general. The specific things I'm thinking of now are:

1. People are living longer, due to medical advances, and
2. Families don't stay together as much as they once did. Many other cultures continue to have extended families living under one roof, while we Americans want "our space" and to live our lives unhindered by the burden of around-the-clock care of aging parents. (I do have several friends who have their elderly parents living with them. They are better people than I could ever be.)

Anyway, when I visited with Mom on Monday, she did recognize me. "This is my little girl!" she told the ladies in the wheelchairs on either side of her in the hall.

"Oh, she looks just like you!" one of them said, and I thanked her. I think my mother is beautiful.

After our usual interaction about practical matters, which are completely lost on her now (I washed and ironed two of your blouses, Mom, and I'm putting them in your closet now. Where is my closet? It's right across from your bed.), I wheeled Mom up to the front lobby where we could visit and share a piece of coffee cake from Starbucks.

I entered her world, as I always do, and complimented her, again, for her landscaping work on the patio (which of course she had nothing to do with) and showed her (again) photographs of her great-granddaughter, Grace, whom she can't fathom, as she struggles to remember even her grandchildren at this point. She can no longer form complete sentences, but speaks in fragments, sometimes apologizing that she can't remember a word, a person, a place.

But suddenly, she smiled at me and said, "I love your hair!"

"Really? I haven't had it this short in years. I'm glad you like it."

"It's very flattering."

Smile. "Thank you, Mom. I really like yours long, in a ponytail, like you wore it when you were young."

This conversation was repeated three or four times, which didn't bother me at all. I could have listened to her praise and compliments all day. They were rare for most of my life. And even though she was talking about something as mundane as a haircut, coming from someone who, when she was "in her right mind," usually criticized me for being fat, having bad hair, etc., this was like healing oil being poured on a wound. At age 58, I was finally receiving praise and approval from my mother.

If this sounds silly to you, you might as well just quit reading this blog post now. Just move along. There's nothing to see here. But if this strikes a chord with you, please keep reading, because it gets better.

As I was about to leave, the sky was getting dark and it began to rain.

"Mom, it's going to be thunder storming, and I need to drive back to Memphis, so I'd better leave soon."

Mom's smile faded, and she reached out, grabbed my hand, held it tightly, closed her eyes and *prayed*:

"Oh, Lord, we ask you to protect Susan as she drives. Take care of her and keep her safe...." She went on and on, for several sentences, speaking with complete clarity.

Tears ran down my face as I listened to my mother, who usually can't speak a full sentence, pray with such beauty and ease. I don't remember my mother ever praying for me, with me, like that. Ever. All the years of verbal and emotional abuse that I suffered from her seemed to melt. Forgiveness gushed from my soul as I listened to her prayer.

When she finished, she opened her eyes, smiled, and kissed me on the lips.

I drove home to Memphis through the rain with no difficulties, and with an unusual peace. When I told my husband the story at home tonight, I said, "Her prayer reminded me of my father, who was an excellent Bible teacher and prayed beautifully."

"She was replaying the tape of your father's prayers," my husband offered. And I wept at his words, picturing my parents doing their daily devotionals together every morning. Dad was eloquent. As an elder in their Presbyterian church, he preached many sermons during interims when they didn't have a pastor. And he led evangelism seminars and taught Sunday School classes. And of course I thought that some day when my mind is struggling to hold on, my own dear husband's prayers will be my salvation.

For all the dysfunction of my family of origin, today I am thankful for this unexpected gift of prayer from my mother's lips. Alzheimer's might be taking her mind, but God still has her heart, as broken and wounded as it is. I pray that He will protect her soul in the coming months and years that she might have left on this earth, and sustain the peace and forgiveness that I experienced today, by His grace.

I Feel So Small
Friday, December 18, 2009

Since my visit with my mother in November, I've been preparing for today's visit with a little less anxiety and a little more peace and joy. It helped that I had a wonderful "lunch reunion" with three old friends from high school first, because we each shared a little bit about our journeys with our aging parents—one who lost her father to Alzheimer's, and another whose mother *and* mother-in-law have just moved in with her and her husband. A terrible consequence of my self-focused anxiety is that I rarely think about how universal our experience is. Thanks to these friends, I arrived at Lakeland Nursing Home with an even greater sense of peace.

Of course I never know, each time I drive down here, if Mom is still going to know me or not, and thankfully, she recognized me again today. (She no longer recognizes any of my children's names or pictures in photographs, and even gets a vague, faraway look when I talk about Daddy.) But today I gave out homemade fudge (Mom's recipe) to all the folks at the nursing home who take care of Mom, and then found her sitting in her wheelchair in the hall near one of the nurses' stations. Her face lit up when she saw me.

I was feeling guilty (a recurring bad daughter theme) because the home was having a door decorating contest and I hadn't done anything for her door, so I was thrilled to find a joyful snowman décor done by the activities director with help from Mom!

Mom's taste memory came back when we shared some fudge, and she seemed happy with her new socks, slippers, and pajamas.

But later, when we were sitting in the lobby, I asked her if the new slipper-boots were comfortable and she said, "Yes. You know, a boy in one of the classes gave me these boots. I don't remember his name, or when he gave them to me, but I said sure I'd love to have them." This was about fifteen minutes after I gave them to her. I wonder if she was thinking of one of the high school students she taught fifty years ago.

I just smiled and said, "I'm so glad you like them!"

We held hands and watched the sunset in the midst of the tall pine trees outside the lobby windows, which are about twenty feet tall. For a while we didn't speak at all, which is very unusual for Mom and me. Twice she just looked at me and said, "I love you." And more than once she said, "I really like it here." And then she looked out the window at the trees and said, "You know, I feel so small. And when I think about dying, I think I'll be okay if I can go to a small place."

"You mean, like Heaven?" I asked. "You know Daddy is there, waiting for us to join him some day. But I don't think of Heaven as being a small place, do you?"

She was quiet for a minute, then struggled with her words, and finally said, "Well, I think my part of it will be small, and I'll be happy there."

Her words reminded me of a sad but powerful conversation a friend told me about last night. The precious twenty-eight-year-old daughter of some friends of ours was in the hospital as a result of seizures she had during the day yesterday. Sara has always been one of God's "innocents," and she told the people with her at the hospital, "I'll be happy to go to Heaven because I won't have Down's Syndrome there." And then she died of a pulmonary embolism. Sara's parents are dear friends of mine from Jackson, and today I'm thinking about how happy she is in Heaven, although I know her family is missing her so much. Sara fought a hard battle, psychologically and spiritually, and in her shadow I'm feeling pretty small. Her funeral will be Monday night at St. Peter Orthodox Church here in Madison, where my goddaughter Mary Allison Callaway's funeral was held eleven years ago. May her memory be eternal.

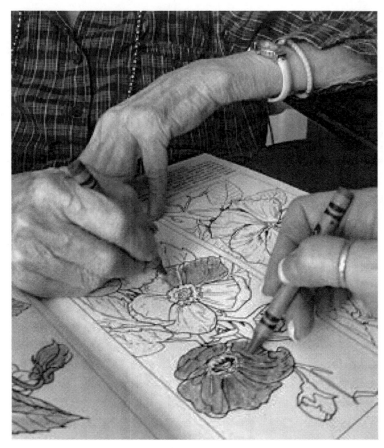

Coloring with Mom
February 25, 2010

Coloring Violets with Effie
Saturday, February 27, 2010

Mom's birthday was February 20, so I sent her a birthday card and wrote inside that I would come visit on February 25. When I arrived at the nursing home on the 25th, I found the card underneath two unopened cards on her bedside table. Having asked the staff many times to please open her cards for her because she has forgotten how, it always saddens me to find these pockets of sunshine hidden inside the darkness of unopened envelopes in her room. I showed her the card I had sent, and opened and helped her read the two others. She looked at all the cards intensely and then said,

"What am I supposed to do with these?"

"Those are birthday cards, Mom. You're just supposed to enjoy them."

"Whose birthday is it?"

"It's *your* birthday, Mom."

She looked around at the walls in her room—her eyes searching for a calendar or some other point of reference—and then asked, "What day is this?"

I explained again about the dates—her actual birthday, and then today's date. And then I helped her open her gifts—two new blouses and camisoles, six pairs of socks, and a new pairs of shoes. Her face lit up as I put the new socks and shoes on her feet and hung her new blouses on the knob of her armoire so I could remind her about them several times during the visit.

Cookies and M&Ms were next. We settled into a quiet conversation as we snacked and enjoyed the view out her windows. The nursing home is right next door to a park, which is shaded by huge pine trees. Being near them always transports me back to my youth and the pine-filled neighborhood where we built our house in 1956. And so I pulled one more thing out of her gift sack—a coloring book and a brand new box of crayons.

Last weekend when I was at Petit Jean State Park with my friend Daphne, I found the book and crayons in the gift shop. The flowers on the cover were beautiful and the coloring pages had instructions about what colors to use on each flower. When I bought it, I thought I'd give it to my goddaughter Sophie, who turned seven this week. But then I remembered how much my mother loves flowers. And that she was very artistic.

But also how much I loved brand new colors and a coloring book. So I pulled it out and asked Mom if she would like to color some flowers with me. At first she said she'd rather just watch, and as I colored the violets purple—her favorite color—and the picture began to come alive, she gushed motherly praise just as any proud young mother would as her little girl colored pictures. I was careful to stay inside the lines because I knew that would please her.

"You are so talented!"

"Thank you, Mommie." Her praise resurrected my childhood name for her. "You taught me how to color, you know. Don't you want to color with me?"

"Okay."

And so she chose an orange crayon and we began to work on the flowers on the next page. There we were—an 82-year-old great-grandmother and her (almost) 59-year-old daughter sharing a delightful time-warp experience, compliments of Alzheimer's.

"You've always been good at art," she said after we finished the second page of flowers. It was as if I was creating a panel for the Sistine Chapel instead of coloring pictures in a children's coloring book with a box of Crayola Crayons.

"You were good at art, too, Mom. And also good at flower arranging. You taught me how to do both."

She set down her crayon and smiled, and then looked wistfully out the window.

"Don't you want to color anymore, Mom?"

"No. I'll just watch you. Can I have another cookie?"

"Sure. They're your birthday cookies—you can have all you want."

"Whose birthday is it?"

And so I explained again and again, and we celebrated the event over and over. My little-girl self taped the pages from the coloring book onto the door of her armoire and basked in the glory of my refrigerator art and the joy of seeing that my mother was proud of me. It had not always been so.

Just as I was about to leave, my friend Sissy Yerger showed up to visit Mom. One of the birthday cards I had opened earlier was from Sissy, so I read the card to Mom again and told her that Sissy had sent it to her. I was trying to help her make a connection, hoping that she would remember Sissy.

She smiled at both of us and then said, "Oh, I know Sissy. She's a friend of my daughter's."

Her words didn't alarm me. They were just a reflection of her choice, that day, to see me as her child, and to speak of her grown-up daughter as if she wasn't there. I'm good with that. My inner child needs all the love she can get from her mother, and she's happy to be the recipient of that love, even when she's 58 years old.

I'll be taking the coloring book back with me on my next visit, hoping that Mom will be happy to see her little girl again.

It will be near my birthday, and of course she hasn't remembered my birthday for several years now. Maybe I'll buy myself another brand new box of Crayolas... maybe even a box of 64 with a built-in sharpener. Why not? I'll be the Birthday Girl, right?

Emotions Outlast the Memories
Wednesday, April 14, 2010

What a blessing I received today from one of my goddaughters, Katherine Thames, who lives in Gulfport, Mississippi. She's a nursing student, and she was listening to NPR's Morning Edition yesterday and heard this short program about how memories can impact the emotions of Alzheimer's patients long after the event is over.

Katherine sent me the link just as I was driving down to Jackson (Mississippi) to visit my 82-year-old mother in the nursing home where she has lived for a year and a half. Justin Feinstein, a graduate student in neuropsychology at the University of Iowa, did a study to prove that events—happy or sad—affect Alzheimer's patients long after they forget the actual event. They showed clips of sad, and then happy, movie scenes to patients, who responded with tears, sadness, or laughter at the time.

Later, even when the patients didn't remember watching the movie scenes, they either expressed sadness they couldn't explain, or an upbeat mood swing after they watched the happy scenes.

The encouraging thing about this is that family and friends of Alzheimer's patients often dread visiting their loved ones because they don't seem to remember the visit. It can be depressing, or feel meaningless. And while I know it isn't meaningless to visit my mother, whether or not she remembers it, it really helps me to know that the things I do with her will cause her happiness long after she forgets the activity. I try to leave her reminders—like taping the picture we color or paint together on the dresser in her room—and I think that helps. Sometimes I send her a photo of us together, from our last visit, in a card the following week.

Today the physical therapist told me that she's been working with Mom on "restorative therapy"—especially walking—for a couple of weeks now. Mom refused to cooperate with physical therapy a year ago after her hip replacement surgery, which is why she is stuck in a wheelchair all day long. But now, she's up and walking (with help) for a few minutes every morning, six days a week. So, I'm sitting in the lobby with Mom this afternoon and I say, "Mom, I'm so glad to hear you've been walking some!"

"Really? I can't remember that." Blank expression on her face.

But then the therapist walks up and says, "Hi, Miss Effie. I see your daughter Susan is here. I've been telling her about how good you're doing with your walking now."

Mom lights up when she sees the therapist and says, "I know you. But I don't remember walking."

So the therapist makes movements, showing what Mom looks like shuffling along, taking baby steps with a walker. Mom smiles and laughs gently. "If you say so."

She doesn't remember that she's been walking every morning, but her overall sense of well-being seems better. I ask if her hip is hurting, or her legs, and she says no. So the movement is beneficial, physically, but I think the personal interaction she has with the physical therapist—a happy, upbeat woman—is what causes her long-term emotional boost.

After spending several hours with Mom today—eating cookies, coloring, painting (with paint pens), sitting outside on the patio looking at the plants, and visiting with various staff and residents, I was preparing to say goodbye. I reminded Mom of some of the things we had done together during those hours, and she had already forgotten about the cookies, asking when we were going to have them. Before listening to this story, I would have been frustrated, but now I'm hopeful that somehow she's going to be on an emotional cookie-high for a while even though she doesn't remember them.

I hope this study encourages more people to visit their loved ones with Alzheimer's. Feinstein says it's best to have short, frequent, "happy" visits. A friend from Mom's church called last week and told me that several people, including her daughter, visit Mom regularly, which I didn't know because Mom never remembers. But I'm hoping that even those short visits are leaving a happy emotional wake.

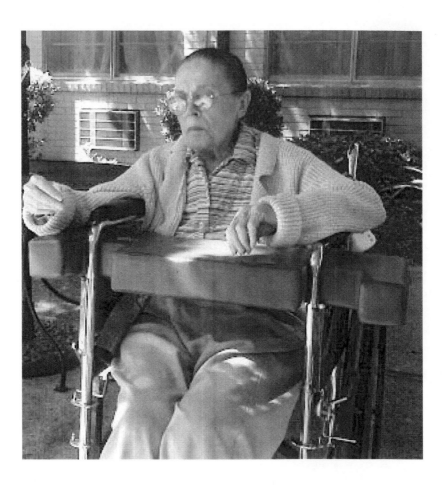

Mother at Lakeland Nursing Home with her lap guard, 2010

A Right to Fall
Tuesday, April 27, 2010

A few weeks ago I got a phone call from the head nurse on the wing of the nursing home where my mother lives. She calls every time a significant change takes place, and sometimes just to let me know of a shift in procedures. This call was to tell me that the physical therapist had been working with Mom again on her walking, in hopes that she wouldn't have to be in a wheelchair all the time. They were removing her "lap guard" and trying her in a new chair, which not only fit her better and allowed her to navigate around the facility better, but it also did not have the large bulky restraint. Instead, it had a seat belt, to "remind her" not to get up and try to walk alone. I was encouraged. For about twenty-four hours.

The next day they called to say it didn't work. Mom quickly figured out how to undo the seatbelt, and would unhook it and try to walk on her own before anyone could prevent her from falling. So they had to put her back in a chair with a lap guard, because she can't figure out how to get it off.

"Why don't you just hook the seat belt behind her?" I asked, thinking she would be more comfortable in a smaller chair without the lap guard.

"Oh, we're not allowed to restrain her in a way that she can't get loose from," the nurse told me. "She has a right to fall."

A right to fall.

Okay, I understand that it takes away her freedom, her independence, her dignity, to be restrained, but I also understand that without some sort of restraint she will surely fall and break her hip again (or worse) and end up in the hospital. But somehow—legally, at least—being in a lap guard, which she could possibly figure out how to remove, isn't actually being restrained.

When I visited Mom today, she didn't mention the lap guard, as she sometimes does. Sometimes she points to it and says, "Is this yours?" or "What am I supposed to do with this?"

I always remind her it's there to keep her from standing up and trying to walk by herself and falling and breaking her hip again. She doesn't seem frustrated by it, thankfully. And they've ordered her a smaller, more comfortable wheelchair with a smaller lap guard, so she should at least be more comfortable.

So, I got to thinking about the legal phrase the nurse used: "She has a right to fall." And I started wondering how and if it would be wrong to take that right from her, the same way we don't let an infant or a small child have full "rights" because they would get hurt. In fact, there are laws about children being in car seats, so they don't have a "right" to be unrestrained in a car. And adults don't have that right either, in states that have seat belt laws.

Today I imagined myself fifteen or twenty years from now, possibly in a nursing home with Alzheimer's. On the one hand, I would want my "freedom" for as long as possible, and depending on my mental state, being "trapped" in a wheelchair with a lap guard might seem awful to me. But I also hope that measures will be taken to prevent me from the pain of falling and breaking something and having to be hospitalized as a result.

I guess freedom comes with risk, and protection comes at a cost.

A New Take on Eldercare
Sunday, August 15, 2010

My daughter and I went to Jackson to visit my mother again on Friday. It was a tough visit for me, for a couple of reasons. First, because Mom was taking a nap when we arrived, which is unusual for her. An aide helped me get her up and dressed so we could wheel her up to the lobby to visit, since her roommate was also napping. It was sobering and humbling to help the aide change mother's diaper and to hear Mother apologize for "making a mess."

"You were napping, Mom." I patted her hand and kissed her forehead. "It's fine, you're all cleaned up now."

Her frown slowly changed to a sleepy smile.

She was excited about the giant cookies we got for her, and for the next two hours the three of us sat in the lobby eating cookies and visiting. It wasn't anything new that she couldn't remember what Beth was doing and asked the same questions over and over. But what was hard was when we got ready to leave. She made the saddest face I've ever seen and said, "You didn't tell me you were leaving so soon!" And nothing we could say would really cheer her up as we hugged and kissed goodbye.

"I'll be back in about two weeks, Mom," didn't dispel her sad expression. She has no concept of time anymore. She just didn't want us to leave.

All weekend I've felt guilty that I'm not there for her more, and even that she has to be in a nursing home at all. She's getting excellent care, and I know it's the best place for her, but it's just hard to shake the feelings of sadness that she is living her last days in such a state of mental and physical deterioration, being cared for by people other than her family.

A friend just shared a link on Facebook to Frederica Mathewes-Green's Ancient Faith Radio podcast from a year ago, "Tender

Love and the Dormition." It's about the death of the Mother of God. I listened to the podcast, and then I read the transcript, and I was struck by several things.

First, Green also has an 82-year-old mother in a nursing home—in a different city from where she lives—so she understands the stress that I feel about my own mother's situation. She also reflects a bit in this podcast on how much work is involved in caring for the elderly, and as a result, how elder abuse and neglect have existed throughout history.

Green's reflections were written last year on this date because of the annual Orthodox celebration of the Dormition (death) of the Mother of God on August 15. I love what she says about the love and care shown for the Mother of God in her old age by the Apostle John, who lived with her and took care of her. Elder care in the first century.

Looking Down
Friday, September 10, 2010

In April I did a post called "A Right to Fall." It was about restraints, and the reasons they aren't used for many patients in wheelchairs. Fortunately, my mother has never figured out how to undo the "lap guard" that slips under the side bars of her wheelchair, and most of the time, the guard doesn't bother her. She doesn't seem to feel "trapped."

When my daughter and I visited Mom in August, she still seemed fairly content in her wheelchair, but she wasn't moving herself around much anymore. In fact, when we wheeled her down the hall to the front lobby to visit, I had to keep reminding her to pick up her feet.

Yesterday's visit was another difficult one for me. When I arrived, I looked for Mom in her usual "place"—parked in the hall with several other residents, right in front of the nurses' station near her room—I couldn't find her. I looked in her room, and she wasn't there, either. I was about to ask one of the aides if Mom was in physical therapy when I spotted her. She was around the corner from her usual spot, parked (with her wheelchair wheels locked) on the other side of a laundry cart, with no one near her to visit with. I approached her slowly, observing that she was slumped over in her wheelchair, reaching down with her right hand, trying to pull herself forward as she held onto the cart next to her. She couldn't move, and no one was paying any attention to her. I fought back the tears as I approached her. She couldn't see me, because she was looking down at the floor.

"Hi, Mom."

She didn't lift her head or let go of the cart, but her eyes looked up at me, and she offered a subtle smile. "Oh, hi."

"I've got some cookies for you—let's go up to the lobby and visit, okay?"

"Cookies?" A bigger smile, but still not lifting her head.

"Yeah, those big chewy ones you like, from McAlister's Deli."

It took us a while to make our way to the front, as she dragged her feet most of the way. She continued to slump forward in her chair. Once I parked her next to one of the couches with a view out the front windows, I got out the cookies.

"Um, what are those?"

"Those are the cookies I brought, Mom. Let's see if I can sit you up straighter so you can eat some with me."

I walked around behind her, placed my arms under hers, and tries to lift her up a bit in her seat. Then I pulled her shoulders back until they almost touched the back of the chair. As soon as I let go, she returned to her slump.

"Mom, look up at the ceiling. You're looking at the floor. Can you look up at me?"

Only her eyes looked up. I physically tried to move her head up and it wouldn't move, so I just sat down on the couch beside her and opened the cookies. I broke off small pieces at a time and handed them to her, wiping the drool from the side of her mouth and her chin as she ate. It has increased quite a bit since my last visit. Finally I had to get up and get some wet paper towels. When I returned, she said, "My back is hurting."

"It's probably because you're slumping down in your chair, Mom." I repeated my earlier efforts, but she continued to return to a slumped position. At one point I noticed her reaching towards the floor (which she couldn't reach) and I asked what she was doing.

"See that?" Her hand shook a little as she pointed at the carpet. There was a tiny speck of cookie. Later she was picking at the fabric of the couch, which had a busy upholstery pattern.

Picking at things is a common behavior among people with dementia. According to one book on Alzheimer's, "Picking is the inexplicable fixation to touch, handle, or work at and remove small items bit by bit...." I've noticed Mom doing this more and more, but at least she's not picking at her skin. Yet.

132

Over the next hour or so, we ate the two large cookies together, bit by bit. Once I cleaned up the table I commented, "Boy, those were good cookies, weren't they?"

"What cookies? Did you bring cookies?"

I'll remember not to mention them after they are gone next time.

Claire, another daughter who was visiting her mother, Emma, sat near us in the lobby, so I introduced myself and Mother. Mother didn't acknowledge her presence, and as Claire and I visited, Mom would occasionally turn her eyes towards me and ask who I was talking to. Claire's mother no longer speaks. She just sits in her wheelchair, looking out the window at the trees.

"Do you live in town?" I ask Claire.

"Yes. I come about twice a week to get her laundry, take it home and wash it, and return it. We usually just sit here by the window for a while—she likes the view."

I fought back tears as I watched this loving daughter sitting with her silent mother. I wondered how long it would be until my visits with Mom looked like this. I thought about the documentary I watched a while back about how "Emotions Outlast the Memories" and I prayed that Emma, and my own mother, could tap those stored emotions—the happy ones—as their memories are being erased.

Before leaving, I tried to find the head nurse to mention my concerns about Mom being "stuck" in the hall alone, and about her slumping, but she was rushing to a meeting, so I waited and called her from Memphis this morning. She had been out of town for a week, and hadn't noticed Mom's slumping yet, but she said she would have her assessed today—probably with a physical therapist.

"It's normal for her to start slumping at this stage—she's probably reaching for things she sees on the floor, even a tiny speck. If she's reached the point where she can't, or won't sit up

133

straight, we might need to get her a reclining chair, to relieve the pain in her back."

I cringed, as I thought about the other residents that I see at the nursing home in reclining chairs, or even in beds permanently.

Leaving the nursing home, I found myself in tears, just overwhelmed with sadness.

I stopped at a favorite watering hole before leaving Jackson, to get a gin and tonic and something to eat. Sitting alone at the bar at Julep's, I felt a little of the pain starting to numb as the Tanqueray and tonic slid down my parched throat. I ordered a sashimi tuna salad and stared at the flat-screen television above the bar. A middle-aged man sat next to me, ordered a martini, and tried to start up a conversation. I wanted to move to a different seat, but I didn't want to be rude.

Right about then three young women came in and sat in a booth near the bar. I recognized their voices and looked up to see two precious young friends whose mothers I had known for over forty years. And then Wisdom, another dear friend's daughter, walked in. They waved me over and we all hugged as Laura and Sarah Anne introduced Wisdom and me to their nursing school friend, Whitney.

Laura and Sarah Anne were best friends with my goddaughter Mary Allison, who was killed by a drunk driver almost twelve years ago. These girls and I share a lot of memories—both joyful and sad. I thought about how wonderful it was to see them studying nursing now, planning to be part of a healing profession. As we drank, chatted, and laughed together, I felt the sadness lift, even as I shared with them the difficulty of my visit with my mother. Friendship and fellowship really do lighten the load, and I'm so thankful for that brief encounter at Julep's.

As I drove home to Memphis in better spirits, I found myself thinking, *I only hope the emotions will outlast the memories.*

Jingle Bells
Excerpt from post on
Sunday, December 5, 2010

On Saturday I made my "Christmas visit" to my mother at the nursing home. I took a gift and dropped it off in the office when I first got there, for "Santa" to give Mom when he hands out gifts to all the residents during a party one day next week. Mom and another resident and I sat in the front lobby for about an hour singing Christmas carols together. Some of them were about Jesus, but some were just "fun" songs like "Jingle Bells" and "We Wish You a Merry Christmas." Mom didn't seem to care which ones we sang. She just had a joy and a smile that I haven't seen on her face in a while.

Alzheimer's is eating away her memory, but it hasn't gotten to the Christmas songs yet. I'm betting they'll be one of the last things to go.

The People in the Box
Friday, January 14, 2011

I drove down to Jackson on Wednesday for my first visit with my mother in the New Year. But first I put together a little post-Christmas gift for her: a digital voice recording photo frame. I printed off a picture of the two of us beside the Christmas tree in the lobby of the nursing home, which I got one of the aides to take when I was there visiting Mom in December. I put it inside the frame, and then recorded a short (six seconds is the limit) message:

"Hi, Mommie. It's Susan. I love you!"

Then I wrote "PUSH & HOLD" and drew an arrow with a Sharpie, pointing to the button.

When I got to town, I stopped by Stein Mart and got Mom a couple pairs of warmer socks (in dark purple, her favorite color), a dark purple sweater, and a long string of giant purple beads. (Long enough that she can see them and "finger them" when she's wearing them.) Then I stopped at McAlister's Deli for her favorite chewy cookies, and I was all set.

When I got inside, I found Mom sitting with a half dozen or more other residents in the dining room, watching the weather on a flat-screen TV on the wall. It was good to see Mom moving around in her wheelchair and not "parked" in a row by the nurses' station near her room. The dining room is spacious and light, and each table has a vase of fresh-cut flowers and a colorful tablecloth.

"Hi, Mommie!"

Her face lit up and she beamed a smile and said, "Well, hello!" (Not, "Hello, *Susan*.")

I sat in an empty chair at the table she had wheeled up to and put my packages down.

"How are you?"

"I'm fine." And then she began to look around the room at the others.

"Is it okay for them to be here, too?"

"Sure it is, Mom. This is the dining room. It's where everyone eats or just visits."

"Everyone? Not just you and me?"

"Everyone who lives here, Mom."

"What about him?" She pointed to a woman at the next table.

"That's a woman, Mom, and yes, she can be here, too."

"He looks familiar."

"Yes, she used to share a room with you. But I don't remember her name."

I showed Mom the sweater and socks, and put the necklace around her neck. She beamed again. "These are beautiful. What are they for?"

"Well, they're for *you*." She fingered the socks and sweater. "Do you want me to put the socks on your feet now? Or do you need the sweater around your shoulders?"

"No, not now. Maybe later."

"I love the necklace," I said, lifting the baubles. "They look like tiny Christmas decorations, don't they?"

"Yes," Mother answered, "I used them for that first, but then I said oh what the heck, and I put them here, on this necklace. Do you like it?"

I just smiled—stayed in her world—and reached for the bag again.

"Okay, well, here's another happy." I pulled the digital picture frame from the bag and showed it to her. More beaming. And then I pointed out the button she's supposed to push to hear the recording, and she pushed it.

"Hi, Mommie. It's Susan. I love you!"

Again, she looked around the room, and then asked, "Are you sure it's okay to have this in here?"

"Sure, but I'll put it in your room with your sweater and socks later, okay?"

"Okay." Serious expression, fingering the frame and pointing to herself, she said, "Who is that?"

"That's *you*, Mommie. When we were visiting by the beautiful Christmas tree in the lobby just before Christmas."

"That doesn't look like me."

"Sure it does. Look at that pretty smile. Although you did close your eyes."

She continued to finger it, but didn't push the button again. So I got out the cookies next.

"Look, Mommie—your favorite cookies from McAlister's Deli."

For the next hour or so we nibbled on the two huge cookies, and she told me over and over how much she loves me. Once or twice we looked up at the television, which was showing the winter snowstorm in Massachusetts. She couldn't figure out what Massachusetts was, and finally said, pointing to the television:

"How did those people get inside there? And... how are they going to get out?"

"Out of *where*, Mommie? You mean out of the snowstorm?"

"No, out of that box on the wall."

She had me with that one. I just couldn't come up with an answer, so I shrugged my shoulders and had another bite of the giant chocolate chip cookie.

Cutting Effie's Hair
Thursday, June 9, 2011

Some people might wonder why I was so nervous about cutting my 83-year-old mother's hair at the nursing home yesterday. It's just a blunt cut, after all. How hard can that be?

It wasn't the physical act that frightened me—I'm actually not bad with a pair of scissors. When I was in sixth grade I cut several friends' hair and even gave a few permanents. It was one of my many entrepreneurial pursuits, and I loved playing beauty parlor.

The fear goes back to a lifetime of verbal and emotional abuse dished out to me by my mother. If you were to meet her now—diminished by Alzheimer's, sweet and mild most of the time—you'd never believe it. But growing up in a home where I was chastised for everything I ate ("That will make you fat!") and how I wore my hair ("It's so flat—it needs some poof!") and how I dressed ("You're not leaving the house in that skirt—it makes you look fat."), you might understand my anxiety over cutting my mother's hair.

She hasn't let anyone cut it for a couple of years now. And this was a Southern lady who got a beauty parlor "do" every week during most of her life, along with a manicure. So when she announced a couple of weeks ago that she wanted me to cut her hair, the aides and nurses cheered me on. (It's hard to wash it and comb out the tangles twice a week.)

Yesterday I arrived with new salon scissors, comb, cape, and brush. Oh, and two new outfits to cheer her up, just in case she was no longer happy for me to cut her hair. One was a peach and white checked blouse with a white camisole and yellow knit capris. The other was a matching set in light blue.

"Oh, where did these come from?"

"I got them for you at Sears, Mom. Do you like them?"

"Oh, I love them—especially this one." She fingered the blue blouse.

I hung them on the knob to her armoire so she could still look at them while we visited in her room and got ready to cut her hair.

I put the cape on her and reminded her that she asked me to cut her hair, and she smiled and said, "Oh, yes! It really needs it."

Since it was so long, I started by simply cutting the ponytail off a few inches below the band.

If you straighten out the ponytail, it measures thirteen inches.

And then I removed the ponytail holder and combed out her hair, which landed in crazy uneven layers along her shoulders. She sat patiently while I trimmed up the layers, taking off more inches and evening up the blunt cut. The view out the windows in her room shows onto a wooded area, which she loves. "Just look at those trees!" she exclaimed while I cut her hair. She never asked how the haircut was going, nor did she ask to see herself in a mirror.

After I was finished, I pulled her hair back up into a ponytail— a short bouncy one now—and smiled at the results.

"How does that feel?"

"I love it!" She still didn't ask for a mirror. *Whew!*

I wheeled her out into the hallway and up by the nurses' station, where we were greeted with more cheers. "Oh, Miss Effie, you look so pretty!" Several of the aides gave me a thumbs-up.

I showed the aides her new clothes, noting which blouses and camisoles went with which knit capris, and she said, "Where did those come from?"

"I brought them to you today, Mom, remember?"

We spent the next hour or so visiting on the patio and in the lobby, sharing a giant chocolate chunk cookie from Starbucks, and just before I left I said, "Well, I hope you enjoy your summer hair cut."

"Oh, did I get my hair cut?"

"Yep. I cut it for you this afternoon. It looks so pretty, and I hope it will be cooler during this hot weather."

"Is it hot today? I'm cold." It was 97 degrees outside, where we had just sat by the fountain on the patio for about fifteen minutes, which was all I could stand of the heat.

"Just be thankful the air-conditioning works here!"

"Can you find my sweater for me?"

"Sure, Mom, it's in your closet with your new clothes."

"New clothes? I don't remember going shopping...."

And that's the way we roll in the world of Alzheimer's, new clothes and haircuts.

I Can't Find My Panties
Sunday, June 26, 2011

When I stopped in Jackson to visit with my mother at the nursing home today, the residents were already sitting at their tables in the dining room, although it was only 11 a.m. The folks in the front half of the room were all watching a local church's worship service on the big-screen television on one wall. But the people (including my mom) in the back half of the room were just sitting around their tables, staring at the white tablecloths or each other, waiting for their lunch. As I looked around the room, it became evident that the residents were seated according to their ability to interact with the world around them. Only the people in the front room were able to follow the television show.

Mother's table was a microcosm of the room at large. Starting at 3 o'clock and working clockwise around her table were these four lovely ladies:

"Helen" smiled as I approached the table and said, "Look, Effie, someone's here to see you!"

I hugged Mom, and watched her smile light up as she said, "What are you doing here?"

"I'm here to visit, Mom. I'm on my way to Fairhope, Alabama, so thought I'd drop by to see you."

"I'm so glad. It's been ages since I saw you."

"Well, it was just a couple of weeks ago, Mom. Remember when I cut your hair?"

"It needs cutting again."

It really just needed washing. They say they wash it twice a week, but I'm not sure.

Continuing around the table we come to "Jane." Mom didn't know her name, and neither did "Helen," but I introduced myself.

"Can you help me?" Jane started pulling off the terry cloth bib the aides had just put on each of the residents at Mom's table and was trying to push her wheelchair away from the table. "I need to go home."

"But it's almost lunch time," I said, replacing her bib.

"I'm not hungry."

"I'm not hungry, either," Helen piped in.

"Me, either," said Mom.

The fourth lady was asleep, and didn't wake up until lunch was served. "That's 'Betty,'" Helen informed me.

Jane took her bib off again and kept tugging at something in her lap. "I can't find my panties."

Mom just stared at her and Helen winked at me. I'm sure she's in diapers, like many in that half of the room.

"Um, lunch will be here soon," was all I could offer, as I helped put her bib back on. Again.

Helen and I exchanged knowing looks and talked about our families. She's from Shreveport, Louisiana, but her family moved to Jackson years ago. I reminded Mom that some of our folks used to live in Shreveport, but neither of us could remember their names. We talked about haircuts and nursing homes and wheelchairs and Alzheimer's (yes) and finally Helen said, "We're all just doing the best we can." And then she smiled this beautiful, peaceful smile.

I looked at Mom, who mirrored Helen's smile. And at Jane, who had quit looking for her panties. And Betty, who finally woke up and ate her meal in silence.

On the drive down to Jackson I had wept quite a bit... just sad from dealing with some of my own difficulties. But after I left Helen and Mom and Jane and Betty at the nursing home in Jackson, I felt my emotions lift a bit on the rest of my drive down to Fairhope. I listened to Neil Diamond singing "Pretty Amazing

Grace" and then Ronnie Dunn singing "We All Bleed Red," and I settled into a place that felt a bit more content in my soul.

As I drove across the bridge over the Mobile Bay and turned down 98 to Fairhope, I remembered childhood summers at Daphne, Alabama (right next to Fairhope, also on the Mobile Bay) and searched for happy memories to outweigh the sad ones. At the end of the day it was Helen's words that kept me afloat: "We're all just doing the best we can."

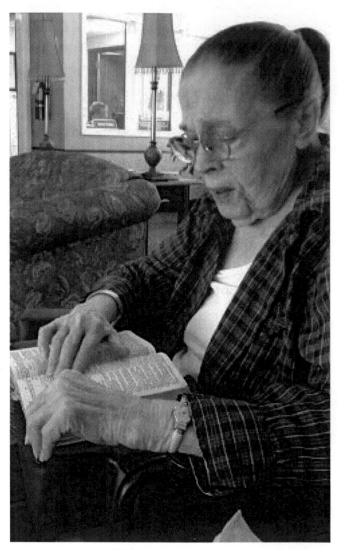

Effie and the 23rd Psalm

The Lord Is My Shepherd
Friday, July 8, 2011

Today I made my bi-monthly visit to my mother. Each visit is a milestone.

The first time I cut her hair.

The first time she didn't remember her grandchildren.

Her transition from verbally abusive mother to loving, complimentary mother.

I have a memoir which was published in *Smith's Six-Word Memoir*: "The upside of Alzheimer's: new mother."

So, today, I took with me two things to my visit with Mom:

A really delicious chocolate chip cookie from Broadstreet Bakery, and a Bible. Specifically, the Bible I received as a gift from my grandmother on Easter back in 1959. I was eight years old. For some reason I thought she might like for me to read to her from the Psalms.

When I got to Psalm 23, she started reciting it from memory as I read, a smile spreading across her face like I haven't seen in years. She was especially lucid when we got to the verses that said, "He leadeth me beside the still waters. He restoreth my soul."

After one recitation, I handed her the Bible, which she fingered lovingly, and then she looked at me and said, "I love you."

I love you, too, Mom.

Disappearing Stories
Friday, September 30, 2011

I was telling a friend about my recent visit with Mom, and she said she has a hard time going to nursing homes. It's so depressing. I remember when my grandmother was in this same nursing home in the 1980s, and my mother would visit her regularly, but I couldn't bring myself to go very often because of how painful it was for me. I regret that so much now, because I know that each of my visits brought her much joy—even if she didn't recognize me or remember that I was there. Because, as I wrote about in April of 2010, "Emotions Outlast the Memories."

The truth is that the visits get harder because Mom's stories are disappearing. She has lost all context for her 83 years of living. I can no longer share photos of her grandchildren and great-grandchildren because she has no idea who they are. She has no emotional response to the photographs and just asks me over and over, "Who is that?" and then says, "I don't remember them." So I've quit showing her photographs. There are lots of pictures of our family on the bulletin board on the wall in her room, and in frames around the room, but I just don't take new ones when I visit now.

We typically sit outside on the patio, where she loves to watch the hummingbirds and flowers, and the other people coming and going through the doors to the lobby. But sometimes, when it's either too hot or too cold on the patio, we sit in the front lobby, where we can see the tall pine trees in the wooded park that separates the nursing home from a baseball park.

"Mom, do you remember all the summers we spent at those baseball fields? Where Mike played Little League, and Dad was a coach?"

"Who is Mike?"

"My brother, your son. He died about three years ago. But we spent so many summers watching him play baseball."

151

"I didn't see him much."

And so I change the subject: "I brought your favorite snack, Mom. Peanut M&Ms and coffee."

Mom enjoyed the entire pack of M&Ms, but at one point the chocolate and nuts were getting stuck in her teeth, and the coffee was gone, so I got a cup of water and offered it to her.

"What's that?" she asked as she took the cup from me.

"It's water, Mom."

"What am I supposed to do with it?"

"Drink some to help wash the peanuts and chocolate out of your teeth."

"Peanuts and chocolate? Oh, I'd love some, but not right now. I've got something stuck in my pockets."

"You mean your teeth, Mom. It's the M&Ms. Here, drink some water."

A few sips of water and she's staring at the trees again. "It's amazing how many people are in there."

"You mean how many trees?"

"They're so tall!" (The pines are probably 75-100 feet tall.)

"Yep. I remember when they weren't so tall, when I was a little girl and we came over here to watch Mike play baseball."

"Who is Mike?"

And so I try for one more story. Mom is wearing a necklace that has souvenir coins from all the trips my dad earned selling life insurance back in the '50s and '60s. Nassau. Hilton Head. New York. Mom went with him to all those exotic-sounding places and they always brought me back souvenirs. When I found this necklace, which was a collection of the commemorative coins from the trips, I thought it would help her remember.

"Look, Mom. These coins remind you of all those wonderful trips Dad earned selling life insurance. Remember going with him to Nassau? It was so beautiful. And so many other wonderful places."

"No, I don't think I got to go with him."

"Sure, you did, Mom. I've got lots of photographs of you and Dad on those trips. Would you like me to bring some on my next visit?"

"Who are you going to visit?"

"You, Mom. You know I drive down from Memphis to visit you a couple of times a month. Like today."

"You drive by yourself? Are you sure that's safe?"

"I'm careful, Mom. In fact, I need to leave now. I'll see you again in a couple of weeks. Want me to bring some more M&Ms?"

"What are M&Ms?"

And so it goes....

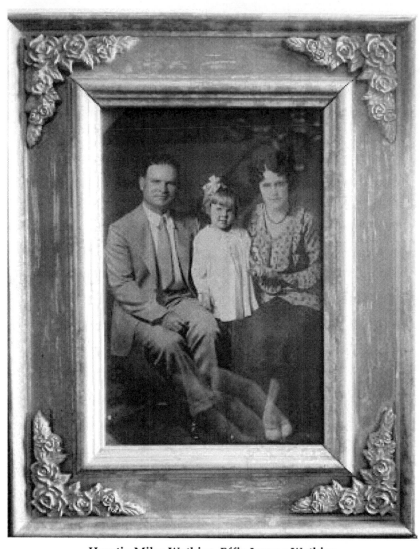

Horatio Miles Watkins, Effie Jeanne Watkins,
and Emma Sue Watkins (circa 1930)
Meridian, Mississippi

Scandal in Mississippi in the 1920s
Monday, February 20, 2012

Today is my mother's 84th birthday. That's her with her parents, Granddaddy and Mamaw (Emma Sue) on the previous page. She's my grandmother who sewed all my clothes until I was about sixteen, and taught me to make homemade yeast rolls and how to fish in the pond at Aunt Lorena's house. And he's the grandfather who molested me when I was about four. He died just before my fifth birthday.

But today I'm thinking about Mom's *real* birthday. You see, a few years ago I was cleaning out some boxes of things I had packed up when I sold her house, and I found her birth certificate. I was about to file it with her other papers when I noticed something odd: *the date on the birth certificate was January 20, 1928, NOT February 20*. I thought it must be a mistake, since we have always celebrated Mom's birthday on February 20.

I scrambled around for her driver's license, and there it was: February 20. I checked other papers, like her Medicare and Blue Cross cards, and they all agreed she was born on February 20.

You'd think I would have just dismissed it as an error, but I couldn't help remembering what she told me years ago, when I asked why her parents moved to Tyler, Texas, just before she was born, instead of staying in Meridian, Mississippi, their hometown. And why they moved back to Meridian a few months after her birth.

"Dad was looking for a better job, so they moved to Texas, and I was born there. After a few months, when the job didn't work out so well, they moved back to Meridian."

With her words hanging in the air, I dug through more boxes until I found her parents' wedding certificate. From JUNE of 1927. If Mom was born on January 20, my grandmother was pregnant with her before they were married. Scandalous in the 1920s. So

155

they simply moved away for a few months and returned to Mississippi with a tiny baby girl (she was small for her age) and lied about her birth date. And her birth certificate actually has a box where you put YES or NO under "LEGITIMATE"! Of course they put "YES." I can't believe it was even an official question on a birth certificate in 1928.

By the time I discovered this, my mother's Alzheimer's was too far progressed for me to talk with her about it. Surely she knew. I wonder when she found out and how she felt about it. I'll never know. And I guess it's a secret she will take to her grave, since she no longer remembers....

Happy Birthday, Mom!

A Practice of Forgetting
Friday, April 13, 2012

I met Robert Leleux in January of 2010 at the 2010 Pulpwood Queens' Girlfriend Weekend in Jefferson, Texas. Along with the Pulpwood Queens' fearless leader, Kathy Patrick, Robert was MC for the weekend, filled with dozens of amazing authors and several hundred members of Pulpwood Queens book clubs nationwide. I was struck by Robert's warmth and compassion when I met him, as well as his humor and joy. And now I understand more about what's behind this "Beautiful Boy." (His first book was titled *The Memoirs of a Beautiful Boy*.)

The Living End: A Memoir of Forgetting and Forgiving, is Robert's latest book, and it's even more powerful than his first. Or maybe it struck me that way because the subject matter hit so close to home—it's about the broken relationship between his mother and his grandmother, and how Alzheimer's (his grandmother's) healed the breach. After reading Robert's exquisite memoir, I realize he has said everything I want to say, and he has said it brilliantly.

When he describes the dissolution of his family life, he says, "This dissolution included Mother taking to drink. (We're Irish.) And it also included Mother shaving her head, and then Krazy Gluing plastic hair to her bald scalp."

And she's not the one with Alzheimer's!

Later in the book, when Robert convinces his mother to meet with his grandmother for the first time in almost forty years, he describes their initial meeting this way:

"It was as though her light was refracted through Alzheimer's, blazing through the cracks of her infirmity. That night, JoAnn might have forgotten the information of her life, her biographical data, but she seemed to remember who she *was*. From her throne-like chair, she aimed all her star quality, all her twinkling, undulating charm, directly at my mother. She beamed and petted and doted upon her daughter, my mother, who seemed flustered and ruffled, thrown off balance by her mother's courtship."

I remember clearly the turning point with my own mother in this regard. I was visiting her in the nursing home a couple of years ago and she kept complimenting everything about me—my hair, my clothes, everything I did. She kept telling everyone around us at the nursing home, "This is my daughter. Isn't she beautiful? She's the best daughter in the world!" Coming from someone who only told me I was fat or my hair was wrong for most of my life, this was at first a bit off-putting. But once I got used to it, it was redemptive.

Robert describes this same phenomenon as he talks about his grandmother and mother's relationship later in the progression of his grandmother's Alzheimer's: "Now that my grandmother had, in a sense, disappeared, she was fully present to my mother for perhaps the first time in their relationship. Now that she was all but unreachable, she was finally available."

I won't give away the story by continuing to quote all my favorite parts of the memoir (which is really just about every page) but I will share Robert's explanation of the title:

"I've always been a person to whom 'forgive and forget' has seemed absurdly unworkable.... since witnessing my grandmother's Alzheimer's, I've begun to wonder whether a small reversal wouldn't better suit humanity. Maybe it would be more practical if forgetting preceded forgiving. Maybe happiness would be more easily achieved if we all made a practice of forgetting."

A practice of forgetting. I'm going to work on that in my own relationships with people when I have a hard time forgiving. And if I follow in my mother's and grandmother's footsteps and end up with Alzheimer's one day, I hope that I will at least by then be able to forget the things I haven't been able to forgive!

Effie and the M&Ms
Tuesday, July 24, 2012

Friends are often asking me how my mother is doing. She's 84 and has Alzheimer's. She's been a resident of Lakeland Nursing Home in Jackson, Mississippi, for almost four years. I visit her about twice a month, and the progression of the disease is sometimes subtle, and other times more obvious. But she always has a big smile on her face and seems content there in her own little world. It's just that her world keeps getting smaller, and her ability to carry out everyday tasks of living is declining.

Last week during my regular visit with Mom, we sat in the lobby where she can look out at the trees and flowers, which she loves. It was too hot to sit on the patio, so we stayed inside, enjoying the view. After a little while, I brought out her "treat." I alternate taking her giant cookies from McAlister's Deli, or M&Ms—her two favorite snacks. Or at least they used to be. But when I showed her the package, she looked confused.

"What's that?

"It's M&Ms, Mom. Your favorite candy."

"Is that so?

"Yep."

I poured a few into a cup. Mom has a slight tremor now and it's easier for her to pick them up from a cup than out of the package. But she just stared at the cup, so I poured three or four of them onto her "lap buddy," which also serves as a makeshift tray for snacks.

"What am I supposed to do with those?" She pointed to the M&Ms, one orange, one blue, one red, and one green.

"You eat them, Mom, like this."

I poured a few into my hand, put them in my mouth and began to chew.

She finally picked them up and put them in her mouth. But no chewing. She just stared at me. After a few seconds, she said, with her mouth full of M&Ms, "They're not moving around in there."

"You have to chew them, Mom."

Once she started chewing, she remembered that she liked them, and eventually ate the whole package. But her brain has already begun to forget simple tasks. I've asked the nurses about her food intake, and she seems to be eating enough to be nourished. She hasn't lost weight and seems healthy, other than her mind. I would imagine that at meals it's more obvious what she's supposed to do with the food on her plate, since everyone else is putting it into their mouths and chewing.

You have to keep a sense of humor about these things. If you are a caregiver yourself, I hope you can also find the humor here, amidst the dark side of this awful disease. And if I find myself in Mom's place one day, I hope someone will be patient with me and remind me to chew my M&Ms.

Tangles and Plaques
Monday, August 13, 2012

I usually don't visit my mother in the nursing home on Saturdays. But this past weekend my niece Aubrey Leigh, who lives in Jackson, wanted to bring her 9-month-old son, Thomas, to visit her grandmother, his great-grandmother. So I scheduled my regular visit for a Saturday. And this time I brought cookies instead of M&Ms.

Maybe Granny Effie often sleeps in on Saturdays, I don't know. But here we were, eager to introduce Mom to her new great-grandson, and she was in bed at 12:30 p.m. Usually she is up, dressed, and has just finished lunch in the dining room by 12:30. The aides tell me she was "kind of tired" this morning and didn't want to get up. I'm actually glad they don't push her when she doesn't want go get up—it encourages me to continue to believe they treat her with respect. But in the nearly four years that Mom has been at the nursing home, this has only happened one other time on a day when I visited, so I was a little flustered, since she had "company" that day.

I was anxious that Thomas would get tired or fussy waiting in the lobby while I helped one of the aides get Mom dressed, into her wheelchair and out into the lobby. Fortunately, he's an easygoing tot and was still in a good humor when I finally pushed Mom up to the visiting area, nearly thirty minutes later.

"Look, Mom—it's your granddaughter, Aubrey Leigh, here to visit you. And her husband, Tommy. And this is Thomas—your great-grandson."

Mom smiles through the tangles and plaques that are gradually killing her brain cells. So, what are tangles and plaques?

The brain has 100 billion nerve cells (neurons) that operate like tiny factories. Alzheimer's disease prevents parts of a cell's factory from running well. As the disease spreads, cells lose their ability to do their jobs and eventually die, causing irreversible changes in the brain.

With this loss of brain cells comes the loss of memory—the stories that make up the fabric of a person's life—as well as the inability to perform everyday life chores.

Tangles and plaques tend to spread through the temporal lobe cortex and hippocampus as Alzheimer's progresses.

Neurofibrillary tangles are twisted fibers of another protein called tau, which build up inside the cells.

Argyrophilic plaques are deposits of a protein fragment called beta-amyloid, which build up in the spaces between nerve cells.

"Whose baby is that?" Mom asks, once I get her wheelchair positioned close to the couches where Tommy, Aubrey Leigh and I are sitting. Thomas is still in his stroller, his big blue eyes glued to Granny Effie.

"He's ours." Aubrey Leigh indicates herself and Tommy.

"Is he your first child?"

"Yep."

"Do you have any other children yet?"

"Not yet," Tommy chimes in—like the sweet and patient man he is.

Aubrey Leigh and I exchange looks. I decide to try again for a memory jog.

"Mom, Aubrey Leigh is Mike's daughter. Remember Mike, your son? Thomas is Mike's grandson—your great-grandson."

Too much information for Granny Effie's tangled cortex.

Aubrey Leigh moves Thomas's stroller closer to Granny Effie, which seems to encourage a little more interaction. When he tosses a toy onto the floor, she lights up.

"There went one of them!" And then his engaging smile and infectious laugh lights up her countenance, if only for a little while.

When Aubrey Leigh gets Thomas out of the stroller, I take the opportunity for some cuddles and hugs—he's a terrific hugger. And then some time on a mat on the floor with a few toys, including the Rebel bear I picked up for him, complete with its own tiny football. Mom seems to enjoy watching him play while I feed her bites of cookies.

I'm glad that Tommy is here—not only for the visit but to serve as official photographer for this first gathering of four generations of my family. I'm wishing my children and grandchildren could see Mom again, but it's difficult with them living in Denver and Savannah. The last time my daughter, Beth, rode down from Memphis to Jackson with me to visit Mom was two years ago, and Mom had already lost whichever cells stored her memories of her other granddaughter.

In Lee Martin's wonderful new book, *Such a Life*, he talks about his mother's and his mother-in-law's decline. At one point he says, of his mother, she "babbles, unable to say what rises up inside her, whether it be love or rage." I can see that Mom is moving in that direction, although she is still able to form sentences at this point.

As my niece and her family prepare to leave, I hold Thomas close to Mom, encouraging her to hug or kiss him, or just to reach out and touch him. "Want to hug Thomas goodbye, Mom?"

"No." Her voice is completely flat.

I move him a little closer and try again. He is all smiles and ready to give and receive love.

"No."

I think of Lee Martin's words that Saturday, as Mother struggles for her own words. I wonder what feelings might be trying to rise up inside her. Aubrey Leigh and I know that for most of my life—and especially my brother's life (her father, who died in 2007)—our mother's words were not kind. In recent years I've come to believe that the verbal abuse she dealt out to Mike and me, and her alcoholism and obsession with weight—hers and mine—were results of emotional, and possibly sexual, abuse by her father. My grandfather, who molested me when I was only four or five years old. This thought has helped me forgive my mother and work towards accepting the childhood I had, such as it was.

Aubrey Leigh's visit, and her eagerness to introduce her son to his great-grandmother—in spite of the past—brought more healing for me. Hopefully, for all of us. Maybe the tangles and plaques can't keep the love from getting through to Mom's heart.

Cousin Reunion, Granny Effie and the Flu
Friday, December 21, 2012

On Wednesday I drove down to Jackson where I was meeting my oldest son, Jonathan. He had driven up from Savannah on his way to spend the holidays in Memphis. We had a lovely lunch with my nieces—his cousins—Aubrey Leigh and Chelsea, at Bon Ami restaurant. I don't think Jon had seen his cousins in about four years. (These are my brother's daughters.) Aubrey Leigh has a son and another child on the way. She's an attorney. Chelsea has an MBA. They both live and work in Jackson. It was great visiting with them. I couldn't help but think about how much Chelsea looks like my mother when she was young. They are all three beautiful women. And my brother, Mike, was a handsome guy.

After lunch Jon and I headed over to the nursing home. He hadn't seen Granny Effie in four years, either. She still pretty much knew who everyone was on that visit.

The annual Christmas party was happening when Jon and I arrived, and I took Mom a new sweater, slippers, and a Christmas necklace and bracelet. I warned Jon that Mom wouldn't know him, but that she was usually cheerful and happy to see anyone.

But when Jon and I arrived, Mom was asleep, sitting up in her wheelchair, in her room. In her nightgown. Her lunch tray was in front of her, and her fingers were stuck in her mashed potatoes. She's almost always dressed and somewhere out in the hall when I arrive. It was about 1:30 p.m.

I called the nurse to come into the room with me, and we couldn't wake Mom up. The nurse had tried to feed her a few minutes earlier. Now she wouldn't open her eyes. She would respond verbally, briefly, and then fall back asleep. I cleaned the potatoes off her fingers and rolled her away from the lunch tray. I put her new slippers on her feet, and put her Christmas jewelry on her. She still wouldn't open her eyes.

So, I stroked her hair and kissed her and held her hand. Jon gave her a kiss and told her Merry Christmas. She never saw him, which makes my heart sad. It's not that she would have remembered that he was there, but I wish they had at least made eye contact.

The nurse said Mom was on meds for flulike symptoms, as well as pain meds for back pain. She had a fall a couple of weeks ago, and is scheduled for an MRI next week. (The x-rays after her fall didn't show anything broken, but this is to follow up.) She's also on Haldol for agitation, which happens often with Alzheimer's.

UPDATE: On Thursday, a nurse called to say that Mom did have the flu, and it would be best if no one visited her for the next fourteen days due to the possibility of spreading those germs. I told her we had already visited on Wednesday (kissed her, etc.) so it was too late.

It was sad to see her like this, but at least she's not in pain. Mom always made Christmas a special time at our house, and I wish I could have made our visit special this week. All I can do is pray that the tangles and plaques in her brain aren't making her sad, and that her back isn't seriously injured from her fall.

Merry Christmas, Mom. I love you.

End-of-Life Issues
Friday, January 4, 2013

Until a few weeks ago, Mom seemed content in her ever-shrinking world — paddling around in her wheelchair at Lakeland Nursing Home, smiling at everyone. And then she had another fall, which escalated to dehydration, a urinary tract infection and E.coli, and eventually pneumonia. So she's been in the hospital for one week today.

The first five days in the hospital, Mom was pretty incoherent. Didn't open her eyes much and was unresponsive to verbal commands and questions. But on Wednesday that changed. Maybe the IV fluids finally helped her wake up, and she began to respond verbally. Up until then, I was thinking this was going to be her swan song. She made it clear that she doesn't want any "extreme measures" and has a DNR order. So, even something as mildly invasive as a PEG (stomach feeding tube) seemed extreme to me.

But with her returned alertness, I was advised by five professionals (three physicians and two priests) — two of whom are related to her — that a PEG would be a compassionate measure, not an extreme one. The PEG tube would hopefully allow her to get enough nutrition that she could get off the IVs and return to the nursing home, where she could be mobile again. One friend, who is a RN, agreed, saying that long-term IVs can be painful. But another doctor told me he doesn't think she will ever eat orally again, which makes the PEG seem a bit more like an extreme measure. Like so many important issues in life — and especially end-of-life issues — nothing here is black and white. So I signed the papers for the PEG tube. As I write these words, Mom is having the procedure done.

I've been here before — first with my father, in 1998. And then with my aunt. Next it was my brother, Mike Johnson, who died six years ago this month. And finally Urania, my dear friend in Memphis who also died in 2007. But each of these folks was in the final stages of cancer when we were facing those end-of-life issues. It was clear that they were dying, and *why* they were dying. With Mom, it's not so clear. Without the PEG, it's possible she would starve to death, which doesn't seem humane. But even with the PEG, she could be bedridden for weeks, months or even years, which also doesn't seem humane. When nothing else causes death, the Alzheimer's patient's system eventually just shuts down because her brain forgets how to run it. I pray for Mother's comfort, and for wisdom in making decisions that are compassionate.

As I walk the halls of Baptist Hospital, I'm struck by the acrylic signs strategically placed on the walls. Each one contains a scripture verse. The one across from me in the waiting room right now says this:

"Those who trust in the Lord for help will find their strength renewed." —Isaiah 40:31

I imagine those words are helpful to friends and family who are visiting loved ones in the hospital. But I don't know if Mom can trust in the Lord in her diminished mental state. Sometimes when I visit her in the nursing home I sing old hymns, and she sings along on some of them. Other times I've recited the 23rd Psalm, and she joins me. So I know that these lifelong elements of her Presbyterian faith are etched on her psyche. Or somewhere. But now when I hold her hand and say a prayer, she just looks at me, through glazed-over eyes. I wonder what she hears. And I hope that God hears.

Mom doesn't know who anyone is anymore. Not even me— although she smiles when she sees me. And once, yesterday, she said, "I love you, too," after I told her I loved her. Usually she just says, "Thank you." I brought a picture of Dad and her up to the hospital from her room at the nursing home and put it in her hands yesterday. She ran her fingers over the picture and said, "That looks like something important." Indeed. They were married for 49 years before cancer took my father at the young age of 68. He was the love of her life, so yes, Mom, this is definitely something important. And today I find myself asking, "What would my father—her spouse of 49 years—do?" It's too late to ask him whether or not to do the PEG, since it's already happening. But other hard decisions may be coming, so tomorrow I think I'll drive out to his grave and sit on the nearby bench under that beautiful tree and have a chat with him. My brother is buried a few feet away. And my precious goddaughter's grave is also nearby. I always feel like I'm surrounded by a great cloud of witnesses when I'm sitting on that bench. Each of them is a hero in one way or another. And I could sure use a hero right about now.

Hi, Honey, I'm Home!
Thursday, January 10, 2013

I'm about to leave Jackson for Memphis this morning, after a week of being here with Mom while she was in the hospital. She returned to the nursing home yesterday afternoon, and to a reception I wasn't prepared for.

It's not that I haven't been pleased with the care Mom has received at Lakeland, because I have. But with her severe decline over the past few weeks—a fall, urinary tract infection, pneumonia, and hospitalization—her Alzheimer's seemed to escalate. At one point I wasn't sure whether or not to have a PEG (stomach feeding tube) put in, but that was done successfully last Friday, and she's tolerating the feedings well. But she has forgotten how to eat, orally. I was able to feed her some soft ice cream the last couple of days, but she doesn't hold the spoon herself. Yet. She's pretty much been in a fog, only responding briefly when I look in her eyes, but not following me with those eyes when I step away. Sleeping a lot, with a glazed-over look.

Mom was evaluated for hospice care on Monday, but she didn't meet the criteria. The hospice nurse said she just didn't have a clear diagnosis of a six-month-or-less life span. Her only option was to return to the nursing home.

My concern was that, while the ambulatory residents at Lakeland seem to get good care, the folks who are bedridden might be ignored. I was so saddened by images (in my head) of Mom lying in her bed with no one paying attention to her. The discharging physician sent recommendations (to Lakeland) that she receive physical and occupational therapy, as well as help from the speech therapist, to try to get her up and around and feeding herself again. I wondered how well the folks at Lakeland would follow up.

So, yesterday afternoon after the ambulance arrived to take Mom back to Lakeland, I followed in my car. As I arrived, the EMTs were transferring her to her bed. I spent a little time cleaning out her closet, putting some new toiletries in her drawers, and chatting with various staff. Finally the EMTs left, and I was alone with Mom in her room. I held her hand, got right in her sight-line, and told her I loved her and that she was "home" now. She didn't respond.

Half a minute later, Lashonda, the head nurse on Mom's wing, was on the other side of Mom's bed, in her face, saying, "Hi, Miss Effie! How are you today?"

The biggest smile I've seen from Mom in days spread across her face and in her strongest voice she boomed out, "Well, hello! I'm fine! How are you?"

Mom recognized Lashonda. In another minute three aides joined Lashonda at her bedside, all fussing over her return like she was a rock star. The nurse checked her all over for skin breaks. Only a small sore on the heel of her right foot. "We'll treat this right away."

"So, what are your plans for helping Mom get up and around again?" I ventured.

"We're going to have her evaluated right away—PT, OT and Speech," Lashonda answered without a pause in the care she was giving Mom.

I backed away from the bed and watched as my mother continued to respond to these familiar caregivers, and tears filled my eyes. What a great team. She really is home.

Love in the Intergenerational Ruins
Friday, January 18, 2013

I made another 400-mile round trip yesterday, to visit my mother. I've been making this drive about twice a month for the past four years. The years my mother has been in the nursing home. Before that, I visited monthly during the three years she spent in assisted living. Seven years of long-distance caregiving. In all those years she has only been in the hospital three times. This last time was a two-week stay, and I was at her side for eight of those days.

Close friends and family who know a bit about the verbal abuse I suffered from my mother for most of my life—especially my adolescent and young adult years, when she was drinking heavily—marvel at my attentive care. "You're such an amazing daughter." Like I have a choice? She's my mother.

The mother I could never please for almost six decades no matter what I did. I could never be skinny enough, fashionable enough, or properly enough coiffed for her approval. And yet, here I am, angsting over every minute detail of her care, especially as the end of her life may be drawing near. I don't want her to be anxious. Or in pain.

When I found her sitting in her wheelchair in the hall yesterday, a sigh of relief escaped my lungs. One of my fears as she returned to the nursing home in such a diminished state a week ago was that she might end up bedridden. And I know this could still be her fate if she lingers in Alzheimer's Hell for many more weeks, months, or years. But there she was—dressed, hair brushed and braided, and her bed made up and room neat and clean. The only problem was that one of the foot holders they had added to her wheelchair seemed to be broken, and her foot wouldn't stay on it as I wheeled her up to the lobby for a visit.

A physical therapist came by and I flagged her down and addressed the problem. She went off in search of a new piece for the chair, saying that this one was broken. Thirty minutes later I found her in physical therapy, busy with another patient, and reminded her. Another therapist promised me they would fix it soon.

"Is the speech pathologist here today? I want to talk with her about what's going on with Mom's oral feeding. The nurse told me they aren't allowed to feed Mom yet due to her risk of aspirating."

"Not today. Call her tomorrow, okay?"

Things aren't perfect in this institution where Mom is spending the final years of her life. But it wasn't perfect in the home she made for me as a child, either. *Ouch*. Did that sound spiteful? Would I have found a way to care for her in my home if she had been a different mother to me? I've asked myself that many times in recent years. There isn't a clear answer. Life is often like that— messy, and unclear.

This morning I read some more of Anne Lamott's wonderful book, *Help, Thanks, Wow: The Three Essential Prayers*. Again, I found comfort and a bit of enlightenment in her words. Not because they are especially brilliant from a spiritual or psychological point of view (although I do believe she's pretty smart and she's learned a lot from what she's been through) but I think more so because of the beauty of her words. It's art. And it soothes and nourishes my soul. And yes, sometimes she helps me find God in the suffering:

> *We find God in our human lives, and that includes the suffering..... We visit those shut-ins whom a higher power seems to have entrusted to our care—various relatives, often aging and possibly annoying, or stricken friends from our church communities, people in jails or mental institutions who might be related to us.... My personal belief is that God... has a certain kind of desperate person in Her care, and assigns that person to some screwed-up soul like you or me, and makes it hard for us to ignore that person's suffering, so we show up even when it is extremely inconvenient or just awful to be there.*

I know that part of Mom's suffering is for my salvation. I hate it, but it's true. I began to forgive her a few years ago, and I keep finding little reminders that God's grace continues to heal me through these difficult times with her now. It seems to be too late to receive anything more from her—she can barely talk now, and doesn't follow my image when I move even a few inches to the left or right of her vision. Only when I'm a few inches from her face does she respond, and then only with one word, "Hi." Nothing more, no matter what words I say. After two hours of this yesterday, I found myself saying, "Mom, are you in there? If you can understand this, I just want to say that I forgive you. And I hope you forgive me. I love you." And in the midst of this I find myself praying. Yes. I think I've prayed more in the past few weeks of Mom's decline than in the past year or more. Pain seems to awaken even my messed up soul to prayer. Lamott nails it again:

> *Domestic pain can be searing, and it is usually what does us in. It's almost indigestible: death, divorce, old age, drugs, brain-damaged children, violence, senility, unfaithfulness.... But grace can be the experience of a second wind.... For us to acknowledge that we have been set free from toxic dependency, from crippling obsession or guilt, that we have been graced with the ability finally to forgive someone, is just plain astonishing.*

And so I find myself embracing Lamott's second of the three essential prayers: *Thanks.* She says that if we are lucky, gratitude becomes a habit:

> *You say "Thank you" when something scary has happened in your beloved and screwed-up family and you all came through (or most of you did), and you have found love in the intergenerational ruins (maybe a lot of love or maybe just enough). Or you can look at what was revealed in the latest mess, and you say thanks for the revelation, because it shows you some truth you needed to know, and that can be so rare in our families.*

Love in the intergenerational ruins. I'm headed to Denver again tomorrow, to spend a week with my daughter, Beth. Beth and her husband are moving to a new apartment and I'm going to help with her daughter, Gabby, and whatever else she needs from me. It fills me with hope to watch Beth with her daughter. She's amazing—full of unselfish love and unrelenting attentiveness. And Gabby is beyond amazing. A child kissed by the angels with physical beauty and intelligence and strength and a quiet and happy spirit. I think she may be God's gift to my daughter, who endured abandonment by her birth mother when she was just over a year old, and then suffered my overbearing ways and lots of craziness during much of her childhood in the very imperfect home into which she was adopted.

Again, Lamott's words say what I'm feeling:

> But if you've been around for a while, you know that much of the time, if you are patient and are paying attention, you will see that God will restore what the locusts have taken away.

I will be 62 in March, so maybe that counts for being around for a while. I'm definitely seeing God restore what the locusts ate. And more and more, I'm able to pray, "Thanks."

There Is a Bridge
Monday, April 15, 2013

Today I'm going to share a link to a video that moved me to tears yesterday. Whether or not you have a loved one with Alzheimer's, if you take a few minutes to watch this video, I think it may change the way you see and communicate with people who are in any kind of diminished state.

Meet Gladys Wilson and Naomi Feill. Naomi grew up in a nursing home, where her father was the administrator and her mother was director of social services. It's been her life's work to communicate with people in various stages of Alzheimer's and other debilitating diseases.

Pay attention to the way Naomi touches Gladys on her cheek, "like a mother does with her child… because the skin remembers."

And the way she uses music to find a bridge to Gladys' past. Instead of being put off by Gladys' repetitive movements, Naomi matches the intensity of her voice with Gladys' movements, connecting with her in a kind of soul dance. It's beautiful.

When I visited with Mom on April 2, she was so much more alert than two weeks earlier. Although my mother's Alzheimer's isn't as advanced as Gladys', I hope that I can build a bridge to her as she slips farther away, using some of Naomi's beautiful wisdom.

(To watch the video, try Googling "There Is a Bridge.")

The Illusion of Control
Friday, September 20, 2013

"Hi, Miss Susan. This is the nurse at Lakeland Nursing Home. I'm calling about your mother."

These calls come fairly often, so I don't usually panic, but sometimes I hold my breath for just a minute.

"Miss Effie is okay, but I wanted to let you know that she has a small skin tear on her right leg, and the doctor ordered some medicine for it, so we're treating it now."

Letting my breath out, I thank the nurse for staying in touch, apologizing again that I haven't been to visit my mother since the end of June because of my accident. She reassures me that Mom is fine and she hopes my recovery is going well. (Note: I was in a serious car wreck in July of 2013, which I wrote about extensively in other posts on my blog, which aren't included in this book.)

A few weeks earlier, another nurse had called and explained that Mom had an infection at the site of her feeding tube, but again, the doctor prescribed meds and she was being treated. Another non-emergency. Another time to breathe in and out. And to thank God that Mom is okay.

Another phone call came this week from a social worker at the nursing home, this time asking me to please sign and return the DNR form that must be renewed annually. This is only the second year I have agreed to this form. Mom's Alzheimer's disease has progressed to the point that she doesn't know who I am, who she is, or where she is. At 85, she doesn't have many other health issues, like heart disease or diabetes. But a sudden "event" could take her life, sparing her more years during which the Alzheimer's will shut down her other bodily functions. She told me, back when she still had her mind, that she did not want to be kept alive on machines. She did not want treatment for cancer or any other fatal illness. Although she doesn't remember telling me that, I remember. And I respect her wishes as we outlined them in her Durable Power of Attorney for Health Care.

Every day I pray that she will not die while I'm housebound due to the wreck. There's really no "emergency" that she might have where my presence would be needed. She is in a skilled nursing facility with access to a hospital, if needed. But how could I make the funeral arrangements and travel to Jackson when I can't even walk? Hopefully I will be mobile in a few more weeks, but this has been my greatest fear since the accident. Sometimes I just worry. But sometimes I remember to pray, and my faith grows when I do that. Faith—the assurance of things hoped for (Hebrews 11:1).

Now that I'm getting close to the point where I can walk, and eventually drive, I'm eager to visit her again. Maybe in October. But until then, I continue to have a great opportunity to exercise faith—to trust that God is in control. Because if there's one thing I'm learning through all of this, it's that I certainly am not.

Don't Touch Me!
Monday, November 11, 2013

Last weekend was my first time to visit my 85-year-old mother in four months, due to my car wreck. For the past five years or so, I've visited her about twice a month from Memphis. I was a little anxious about going so long without seeing her, even though she has Alzheimer's and doesn't know how long it's been. The nurses call me frequently, about every little thing that's going on with her, so it's not her medical care that I was concerned about. It's the fact that she had to go four months without seeing the only person in her family she might still have some recognition of.

My fears were confirmed when her face didn't light up as much when I approached her and said, "Hi, Mommie!" And later, as we were sitting with her on the patio and I tried to straighten her sweater and hug on her a bit and play with her hair, she would say, "Don't touch me!" This was a new development, and it made me sad.

This afternoon I'm stopping in for another visit before returning to Memphis from my weekend in Fairhope. I've brought scissors to trim her hair and a manicure kit to work on her nails, if she will let me. I haven't had time to read up on this new aversion she has developed to be being touched. Is it just part of the process that Alzheimer's works on her psyche? Should I ignore her protests and hug her and rub lotion on her hands, and brush her hair—all actions that I've thought would bring her comfort? Human touch is so important, isn't it? I read a short article that encourages "gentle touching," so I think I'm going to continue that when I see her this afternoon.

MESSAGE FROM YOUR CASE WORKER
Friday, November 22, 2013

I went to bed last night with a feeling of gloom. Not quite doom, but definitely gloom. Why? I had just opened yesterday's mail and found a letter from my mother's Medicaid case worker. The opening line—bold, in all caps, centered at the top of the letter—said:

NOTICE OF ADVERSE ACTION

And two lines down were these words:

Your eligibility will terminate 11/30/2013.

Reason? Your income exceeds the income limit.

The letter went on to say that I must request a hearing by 11/25/2013. That's Monday. And I got the letter yesterday. At the bottom of the letter, centered in bold, all caps, it said:

MESSAGE FROM YOUR CASE WORKER

Now, I've had a pretty good relationship with my mother's Medicaid case worker for the past few years. It was a lengthy and labor-intensive process (with tons of paperwork) to get Mom approved for Medicaid, but when it happened a few years ago, I breathed a huge sigh of relief. Mom's social security and Dad's small state retirement income together weren't enough to pay for her nursing home care. Thankfully Medicaid would make up the difference, which they've been doing for several years now.

Every summer I receive a letter requesting more paperwork to determine her eligibility for another year, and every summer, she is approved. So, this letter really scared me.

I woke up with the letter on my mind. Before coming downstairs for coffee, I stopped by our icon corner to pray. I looked at the reading for today in our Orthodox calendar, and here's the quote I read aloud with my prayers:

Christ is our Friend, our Brother. He is whatever is beautiful and good. He is everything. In Christ there is no gloom, melancholy or introversion, whereas man suffers from various temptations and situations that make him suffer. Christ is joy, life, light, the true light, which makes man glad, makes him fly, makes him see all things, see all people, suffer for all people, and want all people to be with him, close to him.

— Elder Porphyrios the Kapsokalyvite
(For more of Elder Porphyrios' words,
read *Wounded by Love*.)

I asked God to help me as I prepared to phone the case worker. First I gathered up my files from the past two years. I noticed the very small increase in Mom's social security income, and couldn't imagine that it would cause her to be ineligible. I pictured us paying the difference for the remainder of her life and wondered how that would affect our plans as we approach retirement. I wondered if I would need a lawyer for the hearing process if it came to that. And then I picked up the phone and called Medicaid.

In the past it has often taken hours or days for the case worker to return my phone calls, so I was anxious about the deadline for requesting a hearing if it came to that. But the case worker immediately picked up the phone, and I told her why I was calling. Then I held my breath again as she answered:

"Oh, that was an error. You will be receiving another letter soon."

"An error? So Mom is still eligible?"

"Yes, ma'am. You can ignore that letter."

And that was that. No explanation or apology, really. But that's okay, so long as Mom is still eligible.

Yesterday at physical therapy, I was telling my therapist that I had been depressed earlier in the week... struggling with so much pain this far into my recovery from the car wreck. My surgeon, whom I saw last Friday, had mentioned that some people have problems with the internal hardware, and he could go back in and remove some of it from my ankle if I'd like. But he couldn't say for sure that was what was causing the pain. Both my massage therapist and my physical therapist encouraged me to give it a few more months, and helped me with their healing hands and positive words this week.

So, today, I'm going to try to focus on Elder Porphyrios' words—that in Christ there is no gloom, but all light and joy. That Christ makes man fly. Yes, I want to be all light and joy. I want to fly.

How to Pray for Effie
Friday, September 5, 2014

A phone call came from Lakeland just as I was having coffee with a friend here in Memphis. My friend had just asked how Mom was doing, and specifically was I still pleased with her care and is she doing okay with the feeding tube. (Mom no longer takes food or drink orally.) The irony is that the phone call was a nurse at Lakeland telling me that they were sending Mom to the ER because (1) her feeding tube site was infected and leaking, and (2) her bowels were impacted. I suppose that number (1) could happen even with the best of care, but I'm concerned that they were not charting the number (2) situation. No pun intended.

Anyway, I have a cousin who is a pulmonary physician in Jackson and he checked in on Mom yesterday afternoon to assess the situation. After four hours in the ER, they admitted her and did a procedure to repair the feeding tube site. When I spoke with the nurse on her floor last night she said they were doing a culture on the wound site and were treating her with antibiotics. She would be in the hospital for a few days… at least until the infection clears up and the impaction is taken care of. I told the nurse that I had been pleased with Mom's care at the nursing home all these years, and she just said, "Well, they should have been charting her bowel movements and adjusting her intake." Her tone wasn't as judgmental as that sounds, but I'll definitely be talking with the head nurse at Lakeland today.

The first time I visited Mom after my car wreck, she didn't even notice the crutches. I'm heading down to Jackson this morning to be with her for a couple of days. Hopefully she'll heal up and be discharged while I'm there. I say hopefully, but last night I was thinking aloud (to my husband) that it would be fine with me if Jesus decides it's time for Effie to come home to Him and Papaw (my father, who died in 1998) and Mike (my brother, who died in 2007). My husband is an Orthodox priest (and also a physician) and his reply was, "As God wills." This is the Orthodox stand on end-of-life issues. It's not black and white, but it's more about accepting suffering than avoiding it, which is often a difficult pill to swallow.

So, how am I praying for Mom? I'm asking God to have mercy on her. Her quality of life sucks right now, in my opinion. But she's almost always smiling at everyone at the nursing home and endures the indignities of having all her bodily needs met by strangers with quite a bit of grace most of the time. And really, her caregivers are less strangers to her than I am at this point. So I try to pray for them to be compassionate and kind to her, and that she won't be in pain. Thankfully she doesn't usually seem agitated, so maybe the Alzheimer's isn't stealing her peace as it steals her mind. She always smiles when I sing hymns to her or recite or read the Psalms to her. That's my plan for this trip.

P.S. I'm writing this at 9 p.m. Friday night... after a conversation with the head nurse at Lakeland Nursing Home. I discovered that they have been diligent in caring for Mom, but some things just happen when you're 86 and have Alzheimer's. Mom was discharged from the hospital this afternoon and is back at Lakeland. I'll check back in with her tomorrow morning before returning to Memphis. Although I still believe her quality of life sucks, she's decided to rally for now. Or Jesus decided that. Or both.

The War on Aging and the Worried Well
Monday, September 8, 2014

*Note: Be sure to read through to the end to get a last-minute update that brought (happy) tears to my eyes!

If you read my post this past Friday, you know that Mother was in the hospital in Jackson. By the time I got down there to be with her, they were about to discharge her back to the nursing home. They had treated her for the bowel impaction, started antibiotics for the infections around her PEG tube site, and prescribed steroids for her (life-long) asthma, which had gotten worse. She was less alert than she is when I visit her in the nursing home and her situation saddened me greatly. I could only get her to smile by singing, "You Are My Sunshine."

About twenty-four hours after I returned to Memphis, my cousin Jimmy (the pulmonary physician who is treating Mom when she's in the hospital) called with the news that the culture they did around her PEG site turned out to be a resistant strain of staph. She was readmitted to the hospital last night for a two-week course of IV antibiotics. Jimmy and I discussed her options. He is aware of her DNR status and advanced Alzheimer's and her wish for no heroic measures, and how spending two weeks in the hospital increases her confusion and agitation. One option would be to give her an initial dose of the antibiotics IV and then send her back to the nursing home to take the remaining doses orally. But that might not be good enough to prevent the staph from attacking her retinas and she could end up losing much of her eyesight. From a quality of life point of view, having Alzheimer's would be worsened by not being able to see. I agreed that the compassionate choice was the IV antibiotics in the hospital, although I'm sad that Mom has to go through this. I always try to put myself in her place when making these decisions, and I would not want to be blind once I had already lost so much mental capacity.

No one should have to be in the hospital without a caregiver and advocate there with them, if possible. But I'm having some medical issues myself and am waiting to hear from my own physician about possible tests I may need to have done, so I'm not up to driving back down and being with her right now. I have to trust her care to the medical professionals at the hospital—being so thankful for my cousin who will see his Aunt Effie daily and report back to me. This is a blessing I don't take for granted.

All of this has me so anxious I'm having trouble sleeping. I'm worried that I have cancer, although my symptoms could be lots of other things. I'm worried that Mom will suffer unnecessarily. I'm worried that she will die when I'm incapacitated and can't be there to take care of the arrangements. And I'm disappointed that I might have to cancel my week-long trip to Denver next week to be with my children and grandchildren, whom I haven't seen since May. Of course that can be rescheduled, but it's there, another issue within the multi-generational mix.

What am I doing to "handle" my physical and emotional reactions to all of this? Last night I went to Vespers at my church. Today is the Feast of the Nativity of the Theotokos—the Mother of God. It's Mary's birthday. I knew I couldn't go to the service this morning because I would be here waiting to hear back from my GI doctor's office (I left a message over two hours ago and am still waiting). So I went to the Vespers for the feast last night. At times like this the love of the Mother of God can help. After the service, our pastor made a few announcements about members who are in the hospital or sick at home, and then he announced about my mother. Several parishioners came up to me and gave me a hug afterwards and I had a chance to talk with them about my struggles. The human element is often the way I feel God's arms around me, and I'm thankful for those hugs.

This morning as I was waiting for the doctor's office to return my call, I sat on my front porch and enjoyed the amazing "fall is coming" breeze and the beautiful flowers around me while continuing to read Sally Thomason's wonderful book, *The Living*

Spirit of the Crone: Turning Aging Inside Out. I can see Sally's house from my porch and imagine her inside, having coffee and working on her next creative project. Or maybe she's gone to yoga this morning. Sally turned eighty this year, but her mind and body both seem much younger than mine. I'm learning why as I read about the work she did on aging when she was my age.

Chapter Four: The Scientific Paradigm, addresses changes in the medical world and how they are affecting our view of aging. In 1904 the term *gerontology* was coined, followed by *geriatrics* in 1909. As Sally says:

Aging became, and still is, one of many pathologies that science would conquer. The official slogan of the American Academy of Antiaging Medicine, a new medical sub-specialty a group of physicians and scientists founded in 1993, reads as follows: "Aging is not inevitable! The war on aging has begun!"

Lord have mercy! Aging has been seen as a disease, leading many elderly folks to relinquish the care of their health to medical professionals, losing their independence and often getting sicker as a result. A study by Dartmouth Medical School researchers shows that during the 1990s, many more Americans were classified as having hypertension, high cholesterol, diabetes or obesity because the definitions of those diseases were changed. As a result, not only were thousands of people put on medications earlier than many needed them, their minds were reset to consider themselves ill. As Sally quoted in her book:

"The medical profession's term for these people is 'the worried well.'"

The worried well. That's how I feel much of the time. Since allopathic medicine defines aging as a pathology, it's hard not to feel that way! As Sally says,

"Scientific authority not only altered private beliefs and behavior, it shaped public policy."

So, how can I change my outlook? Sally continues:

Aging is not a pathology—a compounding of chronic disease. Aging is a living process that must be understood from both inside (the body/mind/spirit) and outside (within a cultural context), with the realization that there is no clear dividing line between the two. The interworkings are ongoing and extraordinarily complex.

I won't try to share more here, but as I continue reading, I'll be back. If I'm not in a doctor's office tomorrow morning, Sally and I will be having coffee together and discussing this. And I can't wait to have her lead a gathering of women to discuss these topics in a "salon" setting in our home next month.

In the meanwhile, I'm going to try to withdraw from the war on aging and remove myself from the ranks of the worried well. I know this will take prayer, patience, and self-discipline to retrain my mind and my emotions to embrace a healthier view of aging, but that's my goal today.

*NEWS FLASH: Just as I was about to publish this post, I got a text from another hospitalist (and also one from cousin Jimmy) saying that Mom's infection isn't what they initially thought. It's a "skin containment," not a "super bug," and she's being released back to the nursing home today! I am so thankful! And the hospitalist who texted me is the same one who treated Mom when she was in the hospital for two weeks in January of 2013, a lovely woman who actually taught aerobics with me at my parents' store, Phidippides Sports, in Jackson back in the 1980s! Mom is not alone there, and I'm weeping tears of relief and thankfulness right now.

No Memory, No Voice, No Glasses
Monday, October 20, 2014

Before I moved my mother into Lakeland Nursing home early in 2008, she lived at Ridgeland Point Assisted Living for a couple of years. I wrote numerous blog posts about those days, and also about her time in the nursing home. One of those posts was published as an essay in the *Southern Women's Review* in 2010: "The Glasses," which I have included in this collection of essays gleaned from my blog.

I was thinking about that story this morning and decided to write a follow-up. It started last Thursday when I visited Mom in the nursing home. I've been mostly pleased with her care there these past six to seven years, but last week several things concerned me.

When I arrived at Lakeland the halls were fairly empty. Mom is often "parked" in her wheelchair—along with many other residents—right by the nurses' station on her wing. From her perch she can watch the comings and goings and often smiles at everyone. The nurses and aides will smile back and say "Hi, Miss Effie." She seems content in her ever-shrinking world. But last Thursday most of the residents were in the dining hall, listening to a woman who was playing the guitar and singing. The singer had a good voice, and I know my mother would love the live music. I was happy to see the music being provided. But I scanned the room and was disappointed to find that Mom wasn't in there.

I stopped by the nurses' station and asked where she was.

"She's in her room," answered a nurse I hadn't seen before.

I stepped into Mom's room and found her sitting by the window in her wheelchair. She smiled when she saw me, but immediately said, "I'm hot." The sun was shining directly on her face. She had a heavy sweater around her shoulders and neck, and the wheels were locked on her chair, so she couldn't scoot away from the sun. Trapped. While everyone else was in the dining hall listening to music.

After removing her sweater and unlocking her wheels and moving her into the shade, we visited for a few minutes. I had brought her some new clothes, so she watched as I took them from the Stein Mart bag and cut the tags off. First a colorful blouse and three camisoles. Next some soft socks and a new nightgown. Finally some new slippers. She touched all the fabrics and exclaimed with delight over the textures and colors. After I put them in her closet, I noticed that she wasn't wearing her glasses.

"Where are your glasses, Mom?"

She rubbed her eyes (allergies) and looked around the room. "I don't know."

I searched her room and couldn't find them. "I'll be right back."

I headed down the hall and found the nurse—the one I hadn't met before—and asked her about the glasses. "I'll call one of the aides." She didn't bother to look in the room herself, or to apologize.

"I've searched her drawers and all around her bed. She has two pair, so surely you can find one of them. Her vision is completely blurry without them."

The nurse started to walk away when I stopped her. "Wait. I have another question. Why isn't Mom in the dining room listening to the music with the other residents?" An aide had walked up and joined us at this point.

"We take her to activities all the time." Her tone was defensive.

"Mom can't really do most of the 'activities,' due to her Alzheimer's, but she loves music. I'm really sad that she's not in there."

"You can take her down there now."

"It's almost over now, but I want to be sure she's included in the future, and I'm concerned as to why she was left out today."

"Well, your mother can't eat (she has a feeding tube) and they often serve snacks and it would just be mean for her to sit there and watch everyone else eat."

"Mom doesn't even know what food is, and it doesn't bother her to watch people eat. She still goes to meals just to be around people." The aide nodded but offered no reply. "I'd like to speak with a social worker about this, please."

"I'll page one for you."

"Okay, I'll be in Mom's room."

I went back into Mom's room and continued to search for her glasses. No one came to help me, and no social worker showed up. Finally I needed to leave to drive back to Memphis. When I got home I called and asked for the social worker. The director of social services wasn't there but they put me through to a social worker. I told her my concerns, and she said she would be sure Mom was taken to any music events in the future. Then I asked about her glasses.

"I've got some here in my drawer that have been turned in," she said.

"Great. Why don't you take a picture of them and text it to me. I would recognize them."

She texted me pictures of two pairs. They weren't Mom's glasses. I decided to send her a picture of Mom wearing her glasses, to help her recognize them.

"I'll check the other glasses in my drawer and see if they match."

She never called me back. That was last Friday. I was out of town Saturday and Sunday but I called this morning to see if they had found her glasses. I got the social worker's voice mail. So I asked for the nurses' station. A nurse answered and I told her my concerns. She put me on hold to go and see if Mom had her glasses on this morning. No. And she couldn't find them in her room. She apologized and said she would search the rooms of others who wear glasses. Maybe an aide put them in the wrong room after taking the residents to the shower or something. I told her about my concerns about the music and Mom being "trapped" in her room and all that. She was sweet and apologetic. I'm hoping this was an isolated incident.

It's so hard when someone is completely helpless and dependent upon the kindness of others for their care. An 86-year-old woman with Alzheimer's and bad eyesight and no "voice" to speak up for herself. I'm trying to be her advocate, and hopefully I found help with this sweet nurse this morning. She's going to call me this afternoon and let me know about the glasses. And she's going to talk with others about being sure Mom is taken to musical events in the future. I'm much more at peace after talking with her. Just praying they find her glasses....

A happy update: at 11:15 the nurse called me back to say they found her glasses! She has them on and is "happily wheeling herself up and down the hall again." I am so thankful.

Caring For Mom and Dad
Monday, May 11, 2015

On our way home from Seagrove Beach, Florida, on Saturday, my husband and I stopped in Jackson to visit my mother. It was the day before Mother's Day. I usually visit her about once a month now, making the 400-mile round trip in one day, with an hour-long visit while I'm there. That may not sound like much, but at this advanced stage of Alzheimer's, my caregiving is different than it was when she was living alone in her home, and later when she was in assisted living. Due to her advanced Alzheimer's, she no longer knows who anyone is and is completely dependent upon the nurses and aides for her care.

PBS ran a special on Mother's Day—*Caring For Mom And Dad*. The documentary shows several different family situations where an adult child is spending a minimum of 20+ hours a week caring for aging parents. For many it is a 24/7 job.

The average age of these caregivers is 49. I began helping Mom in 1998, when my father died. Mom was 70 and I was 47. Now Mom is 87 and I'm 64.

Sixty-one percent of the caregivers in the PBS film are employed, often "sandwich moms" raising a family, working full time, and caring for one or more aging parents.

Since 1950 we've added more than a decade to the life-span of most Americans. Seventy-six million baby boomers are all going to get old at the same time. Seventy percent of adults 65 and older will need some form of long-term care. How will our children care for us? What is the government doing to help prepare for this? These are a few of the questions addressed in the PBS special.

Although my mother has been in a nursing home since late 2008, for ten years before that I was more involved in her day-to-day living: taking care of her finances, eventually cleaning out her house and selling her house and car and moving her to assisted living. Being with her through several hospitalizations. All of this while living 200 miles away and making monthly or sometimes weekly trips to help her. I have so much to be thankful for—especially that she agreed to make me her Durable Power of Attorney and put me on her bank accounts before her dementia had progressed to the point where she wouldn't have been able to do so. I'm also extremely thankful that Medicaid stepped in when her own finances ran out a few years ago.

One daughter in the film said she couldn't imagine not taking care of her mother at home. She couldn't imagine putting her in a home. She would feel like a bad daughter.

It's hard to hear those words and not feel guilty at times. But the truth is:

1. I cannot physically care for my mother 24/7, since she is in a wheelchair, wears diapers, and has a feeding tube. She cannot do anything for herself.

2. Medicaid won't pay for the in-home care she needs, but it does pay for nursing home care.

I have two friends who cared for one of their aging parents at home for many years. Several other friends are in the throes of caregiving decisions right now—some are helping their parents in independent living, others in assisted or nursing homes.

Each caregiver's situation is different, and we all need to do the best we can and try not to be too hard on ourselves. It's difficult enough caring for dependent parents without the added guilt trip. The main thing is to communicate our love for them no matter what level of caregiving we are involved in.

Mother was speaking non-stop nonsense when we stopped to see her on Saturday. She talked about the "trouble" and how "they're trying to fix it." She talked about "the colors over there" (pointing towards her window) and how they "just go here and there all the time." She had no idea who we were, or what Mother's Day is. But I rubbed her hands, sang to her, kissed her several times and kept telling her I loved her. She smiled a lot and returned the kisses. When we got ready to leave (which is always difficult) she just waved and smiled.

But out in the hall a woman kept asking us to please call her daughter to come get her out of there. The urgency and confusion on her face was gut-wrenching. I don't know her daughter, but I choose to believe that she, too, is doing the best she can.

Tangles and Plaques, the Book
Monday, October 5, 2015

On November 24, 2007, I wrote my first blog post about my mother. Today's post will be my 54th. While driving to and from Jackson to visit Mom this past Friday, I decided what my next book project will be. I'm going to put together a collection of essays from those blog posts. I've got 47,651 words in these posts so far—just the right size for a small book. Of course the word count could shrink or grow with editing, but I'm thinking this could be a good book. Working title is *Tangles and Plaques*, which comes from my post on August 13, 2012, "Tangles and Plaques."

So what about my visit on Friday?

When I arrived I went to Mother's room and someone else was in her bed! I freaked out and went running to the nurses' station to ask where my mother was. The nurse at the desk calmly replied, "Room 208." But on the way to room 208 I found Mom, in her wheelchair in the hallway. She was fine, so I left her briefly to go look in room 208. There was all her stuff—her pictures, her clothes, everything. Why hadn't someone told me about this move? The last time they moved her they called me and asked if it was okay and everything. I was a bit upset, and I went to the front office and asked to speak to a social worker.

Meanwhile I wheeled Mom up to the front lobby where we could see outdoors while we visited. She looked so much older—like she had aged quite a bit in the few weeks since I had seen her. For the first time ever, when I sang "You Are My Sunshine" and "Amazing Grace," she didn't sing along or even smile. When I would finish a song she would say, with no emotion, "That's nice." It broke my heart to see her this much more diminished. And yet still here. (Remember when I said I asked Jesus why she was still here? I still don't have an answer.)

And then the social worker joined us in the lobby and reminded me that she had called me on the phone about moving

Mother to another room. As she spoke about the details of the call, it began to come back to me. Vaguely at first, and then more vividly. I apologized to her and said something about me having a senior moment. But it was so scary. Because this is how it all started for Mom, when she was not a whole lot older than me.

The event confirmed my desire to publish this book while I still can. I don't mean to sound alarmist, but I know that a project like this could easily take 2-3 years, and I've also got a novel and an anthology, which I'm editing, in the works. Do I have the mental health to pull this off? I'm determined to try.

Before the tangles and plaques get me.

Tangles and Plaques, Part II
Monday, October 12, 2015

Since last Monday's post, *"Plaques and Tangles,"* I've had many opportunities to continue my focus on Alzheimer's—not only my mother's, but my friend Sissy's—and also the possibility that this will be my fate. Sissy was only 73 when she died last week. That's about the age my mother was when her cognitive impairment began to increase enough that I started taking care of her finances and we began considering assisted living. I am so thankful that Sissy was spared the years of decline my mother—now eighty-seven—is still experiencing.

A dear friend who is completely alert in her eighties encouraged me to quit dwelling on it so much, saying that I could "think myself sick." There's wisdom in her words, I know, but it's really hard not to think about this. Especially with regular visits to my mother in the nursing home, and now as I work on editing those blog posts and turning them into essays for a potential book.

One reader left this comment on last Monday's post: (This is only part of her comment.)

> *As someone with a family history, I understand your fears. It's certainly entirely possible that the phone conversation slipped your mind due to fatigue, pain, busy-ness, distractions, etc. Obviously, your fear is that it is an early symptom of Alzheimer's, which is a valid concern. Do you have access to a gerontologist or other specialist who could do a screening? (I suggest a specialist because in my family's experience primary care doctors often miss early signs.) If the screening results show nothing, it can set your mind at ease. If there are early signs, you can begin treatment to slow progression so that you can continue your three(!) book projects.*

You know, I never had my mother screened for Alzheimer's. I just saw it happening and dealt with each stage as it progressed. Well, she was "screened" by her internal medicine physician early

203

on, but she always passed those simple memory tests. I remember sitting in the doctor's office while this was going on and thinking, "But you don't see how diminished her functioning is outside of this room." So, I do know that if I decide to be screened, I'll go to a specialist who will do more than ask me who the President is and what street I live on and to count backwards from ten.

I'll be 65 next March, so I've been receiving lots of information about Medicare. And I just read this article on NPR, "Medicare Pays for Alzheimer's Screening, But Do You Want to Know?" One argument FOR early screening is to establish a baseline for comparison. But there's so much that's unknown at this point. November 1-7 is actually National Memory Screening Week, an initiative of the Alzheimer's Foundation of America. There are actually two sites in the Memphis area offering free screening that week. But I haven't looked into how extensive the tests are. Not sure if I'm going to or not. Stay tuned, and thanks always for reading and commenting.

Mom's Unsung Heroes
Monday, October 19, 2015

This is my 56th post about my mother since I began my blog in 2007. Most of those posts are about *her*—her unfortunate decline with dementia and Alzheimer's. Today's post is about her caregivers. I rarely write about the good care my mother receives at Lakeland Nursing Home in Jackson, Mississippi, but her nurses and aides and physical therapists and activities directors and social workers really are her unsung heroes.

In the past week alone I've received five phone calls from various people who are taking care of her. First a nurse called to let me know the doctor had changed the dose on her psychotropic medicine to help with agitation·and sleep. They call and let me know about everything they do for her that involves her treatment.

Next I got a call that Mom had pulled her PEG tube out of her stomach (again) and they would send her to the hospital to have it put back in. Of course she has no idea what it is, and although they keep a lot of padding over it, when she can't sleep or gets agitated she picks at it until she finally pulls it out. I'm amazed that this is only the second time she's done this in the nearly two years she's had the feeding tube. So, they call me when she leaves for the hospital, then a nurse at the hospital calls to get my permission for the procedure, and then they call me when she returns to Lakeland, doing just fine.

The next day I got a call from the activities director. She wanted to ask me which activities I thought meant the most to my mother. She's way past being able to play bingo or follow a television show, but she still responds to music, so I suggested they be sure and take her into the dining room whenever there's any music. And on Fridays some people from Covenant Presbyterian Church (the church my parents helped start in the

1950s) come and lead the singing and do a little devotional. I'm sure the hymns and words must resonate with her 87-year-old Presbyterian soul. We discussed a few more things that might connect with Mom at this stage of her Alzheimer's.

So, this is just a big THANK YOU to Mom's angels at Lakeland. Her unsung heroes.

Life in the Shadows
Monday, November 30, 2015

As I continue editing my blog posts about caregiving for my mother, who has Alzheimer's—hoping to turn them into a collection of essays for publication—I'm also reading an inspirational book. *The New York Times* bestseller *Turn of Mind*, by Alice LaPlante, is a fictional account of an orthopedic surgeon's decline with Alzheimer's. It's also a murder mystery. Brilliant book.

Since I've titled my essay collection *Tangles and Plaques*, I was excited to see LaPlante's use of those terms in her book:

> *This half state. Life in the shadows. As the neurofibrillary tangles proliferate, as the neuritic plaques harden, as synapses cease to fire and my mind rots out, I remain aware. An unanesthetized patient.... Every death of every cell pricks me where I am most tender.*

Ouch. LaPlante's book is difficult to read, but I can't put it down. Especially since she's combined the psychological aspects with a murder mystery. Who killed Jennifer's best friend, Amanda?

It's also interesting to me that LaPlante's protagonist, Dr. Jennifer White, was raised as a Catholic, and her most prized possession is an icon of Saint Rita of Cascia, the patron saint of lost causes.

Alzheimer's. Murder mystery. Icons. I'm only halfway through the book, but every page contains treasures.

Making Memories
Friday, December 11, 2015

If you read my blog regularly, you know that I have as many unhappy as happy memories of my childhood—mostly because my mother was verbally and emotionally abusive much of my life. I've written fifty-eight blog posts (usually in my "Mental Health Monday" series) about caregiving for Mom since 2007. When I visited her this week on my way to and from Fairhope, Alabama, I found her slipping ever farther away, her mind tangled with advanced Alzheimer's disease. I've forgiven her and come to understand more about why she was the way she was in the past few years, leaving me with more compassion for her, and sending me on a search for more happy memories, especially during this Christmas season.

This morning I made fudge for a cookie swap I'm going to tomorrow morning. Watching the chocolaty mixture develop that shine as it melted and blended together, smelling the seductive aroma of the butter and chocolate, tasting the warm mixture as I spread it over sheets of waxed paper, took me back to memories of making fudge with my mother many times in my childhood. It was one of my favorite activities.

Every time Mom and I made fudge, she would tell me about her favorite childhood memory—making pecan divinity with her mother. Mom was a sickly child, with asthma that kept her inside a lot, especially during the winter months, even in Meridian, Mississippi. To keep her entertained, Mamaw (her mother) would let her help make pecan divinity. If you've never had (a homemade version of) this confection, you've missed a real treat. I understand why they call it divinity—it is truly divine! But for whatever reason, Mom and I never made it. But we made outstanding fudge.

I made sugar cookies with my own children—the kind you decorate with sprinkles and frosting and candies. And I love doing this with my granddaughters when we visit them in Denver, as we'll be doing again this Christmas. Oh, and my daughter-in-law bought those little gingerbread house kits for me to make with her girls last year, which is another fun tradition.

I hope that however dysfunctional (or not) your childhood home was, you can find some good memories to focus on during this Christmas season. My eyes are filled with tears and a smile is spreading across my face as I type these words. I'm so thankful to my grandmother and my mother for these nurturing memories. No, my life hasn't been perfect, but making fudge this morning has brought to mind something good: three generations of sweetness. I'm only sorry that Mom can no longer eat fudge or divinity. I feel sure the flavors of these memories could burst through some of those tangles and plaques.

Prayer Cards for Effie
Friday, January 15, 2016

When I was visiting my mother in the nursing home this past Monday, I found several "prayer cards" in a drawer of the table by her bed—notes from a group of people at Covenant Presbyterian Church in Jackson, Mississippi—the church my parents helped establish in the 1950s—who get together every Monday (or so the dates seem to say) to pray for people. I found cards dating back to January of 2015, some opened, others still in sealed envelopes.

Mom hasn't been able to read mail for a couple of years. She no longer understands what it is, and of course she doesn't recognize the names of the people who send her cards and letters. But the love and prayers behind the cards are such a blessing to me.

Yesterday I read through those cards and wrote thank-you notes to several folks whose names I recognized. What a joy to see Jeffie Carter—who taught me in the second grade at Spann Elementary School—amongst them. Jeffie must be in her late '80s or early '90s by now. She was my very favorite teacher of all time. Also amongst the names were Linda and Auburn Lambeth. Auburn was my Sunday School teacher at least one year at Covenant. Dr. Boyd Shaw—the compassionate physician I called upon during the final days and hours of my father's life when the hospice nurses couldn't get Dad's doctor to prescribe more morphine. Ernie Strahan, Richard Coker, and Virginia Brock's names were also there—other founding members of the church from over fifty years ago.

As I read over the names, I thought about the fact that my mother would be one of those people gathering to pray on Mondays, and signing her name to the cards being mailed out, if she could. How tragic that she's the one in the nursing home instead—no longer able to read the cards and remember these people she's known for so long.

When I wrote my thank-you notes to several of these people, I told them that their prayers were like hidden treasures, so valuable and yet unseen by most people. But not God. I believe He hears their prayers, and that somehow—in a mystery—my mother is comforted by them.

Epilogue
No More Tangles and Plaques
Monday, May 23, 2016

I've been blogging about my mother—and my long-distance caregiving for her as her Alzheimer's advanced—since 2007. Today I'm thankful to share the news that her struggle with this awful disease is over. Mother died Sunday, May 22, at 1:20 p.m. at St. Dominic Hospital in Jackson, Mississippi. She had wonderful assistance from the caring nurses and doctors at St. Dominic, and also from Hospice Ministries the final three days of her life. And I had wonderful help from our oldest son, Jon, our niece Aubrey Leigh, and several friends who spent time with Mom in the hospital. Many blessings.

My first cousin Jimmy Jones is a pulmonary physician in Jackson, and takes care of many elderly patients. I was blessed to have him involved in Mom's care. He is very familiar with end-of-life issues. Jimmy shared an article with me by Harvard physician Atul Gawande. It's lengthy but well worth the read: "Letting Go: What Should Medicine Do When It Can't Save You?"

We are burying Mom today at Natchez Trace Memorial Park Cemetery, where we buried my brother, my father, and a dear friend's daughter. Their graves are just a few feet apart on a little hill with a beautiful tree and a bench for sitting and praying or remembering these loved ones. My husband will officiate the funeral—which was Mom's request to him many years ago. I'll close this post with the obituary which appears in Jackson's *Clarion Ledger* newspaper today. I love you, Mom. May God grant you Paradise.

Effie Watkins Johnson

Jackson, MS

Effie Jeanne Watkins Johnson of Jackson, Mississippi, died on May 22 at the age of 88. She was preceded in death by her husband, W. E. (Bill) Johnson, Jr., and her son, Michael Johnson, both of Jackson. She is survived by her daughter, Susan Johnson Cushman, of Memphis; grandchildren Jonathan Cushman of New Orleans, Jason Cushman and Elizabeth Cushman Davis of Denver, Aubrey Leigh Johnson Goodwin of Jackson, and Chelsea Boothe Bennett of Atlanta; and six great-grandchildren.

Mrs. Johnson was born on February 20, 1928, in Tyler, Texas, to Emma Sue Covington Watkins and Horatio Miles Watkins. She grew up in Meridian, Mississippi, and graduated from Mississippi State College for Women. She married Bill Johnson in 1948 and taught at Central High School and as a substitute teacher in the Jackson Public Schools. She and her husband were charter members of Covenant Presbyterian Church. After Mr. Johnson's retirement from U.S.F. & G. Insurance Company in 1982, the couple opened Bill Johnson's Phidippides Sports, which they operated together until its closing in 1997, one year prior to Mr. Johnson's death. Mrs. Johnson had been a resident at Lakeland Nursing Home since 2008 as a result of Alzheimer's Disease.

One legacy Mrs. Johnson left her children was the tradition she and Mr. Johnson had of greeting one another every morning with "This is the day the Lord has made!" and the response, "Let us rejoice and be glad in it." After his death, she would say the greeting and response to her husband as she looked at a picture of the two of them in her bedroom, having a firm conviction that he was very much alive in Heaven. Her daughter and son-in-law have continued the tradition to this day.

Visitation will be at Natchez Trace Funeral Home at 10 a.m. on Tuesday, May 24, followed by a service in the chapel at 11 a.m. and the interment at Natchez Trace Cemetery, 759 US-51, Madison, MS 39110. Memorials may be made to the Alzheimer's Foundation of America.

Ode to Granny Effie: A Grandson's Tribute
By Jason Cushman

(Note: Our 35-year-old son Jason wrote this a couple of days before his grandmother died, when she was in the hospital with hospice care. My husband, an ordained Orthodox priest, read it as part of his homily at Mother's funeral. Jason was adopted from South Korea when he was almost three.)

What do I remember about you?

I remember a woman that was always happy. Always so polite and hospitable. I could instantly see where my mother got her manners, manners she then passed on to her children. "Southern Hospitality" is more than just a phrase. It has deep meaning in the way we treat other people and no one was more loving than you. I don't remember ever hearing you say a word in anger. Not once. But I also can't remember Papaw saying a word in anger either... so perhaps that is just how all grandkids are supposed to remember the elders they love and respect.

I remember feeling different, but never feeling like I was "adopted" in Jackson, Mississippi. This is no small thing because I was continuously reminded of that later in life. There are frozen mental images of Phidippides, the retail sports store my grandparents owned from 1982-1997—clothes on racks, a back room with a play area, and a workout room. I don't know what is my memory and what are figments of my imagination, but in most of them you are smiling. You are there offering us a peppermint piece of gum, the square ones with the liquid in the middle.

They are great memories because I remember you in them. I imagine, although I thankfully can't remember, that my year prior to arriving in Jackson was not the happiest time in my life. I imagine a lot of the happiness I found was due to your kindness, that of you and your husband. The gift of your daughter, my

215

mother, and my parents' gift in turn in adopting me. Of giving me the life that although sometimes has been dark, now is a light unto itself with my wife and children, which I never thought I would have. I hope you aren't in pain right now. I hope you know we love you.

Acknowledgments

I probably would never have considered putting together this collection of essays without the support of so many loyal readers of my blog, *Pen and Palette*, which I started in 2007. And although the sixty blog posts about my mother that now appear as essays in this book comprise a small percentage of the nearly 1,400 posts I had published on *Pen and Palette* when this book went to press, they almost always garnered more comments on the blog and more "likes" on Facebook than my posts about other subjects. High school friends like Mary Eckert Zimmerman and Kathy Moore Kerr often left encouraging comments, as did many others who were also dealing with aging parents, some with Alzheimer's. My best friend here in Memphis, Deb Davidson Mashburn, frequently told me how much my words blessed her. New friends from social media circles began following the blog, also offering regular comments. Most of those readers were baby boomers like me, the generation most immediately affected by the onslaught of Alzheimer's disease.

But it was someone from my children's generation who planted the seed for this book, whether intentional or not. I am so thankful to Erin Mashburn Moulton for telling me over and over again that my posts about my mother represented the best of my writing. Thank you, Erin!

Members of my writing group—Suzanne Henley, Ellen Morris Prewitt, Emma Connolly, Blake Burr, Sybil McBeth, Melinda Shoaf, Dan Stringfellow, Sandi Butler Hughes, Joseph Hawes, and Tom Carlson—gave valuable feedback on parts of the book, as did my friend, the author Sally Thomason.

I also want to thank my husband of forty-six years for helping me navigate this journey with my mother. And our children, Jonathan, Jason and Beth, and my niece Aubrey Leigh, for their love and devotion to their grandmother, even in those latter years when she no longer knew who they were. Their long-distance trips to visit her in the nursing home in Mississippi—and to bring great-grandchildren to meet her when possible—often fed my spirit when I needed encouragement, and I'm sure Granny Effie felt your love at some level.

One final word of thanks—and this one really isn't about the book, but it's about the journey—goes to my first cousin Jimmy Jones, the physician who was always there for Mom each time she was hospitalized. And during her final stay at St. Dominic Hospital, it was her nephew Jimmy who helped us navigate the difficult end-of-life issues. We were so blessed to have you there. This book—and Mom's life—would not have ended as peacefully without you.